Pediatric Human Immunodeficiency Virus (HIV) Infection

A Compendium of AAP Guidelines on Pediatric HIV Infection

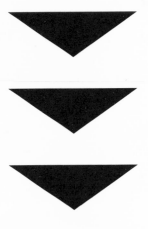

American Academy of Pediatrics

Pediatric Human Immunodeficiency Virus (HIV) Infection

A Compendium of AAP Guidelines on Pediatric HIV Infection

A compilation of AAP policy statements
and excerpts from manuals published
through August 1994

American Academy of Pediatrics
141 Northwest Point Blvd
Elk Grove Village, IL 60007

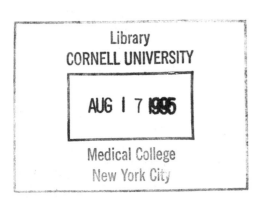
ISBN No. 0-910761-51-5

MA0065

Quantity prices on request. Address all inquiries to:
American Academy of Pediatrics, PO Box 927,
141 Northwest Point Blvd, Elk Grove Village, IL 60009-0927

The recommendations in this publication do not indicate an exclusive course
of treatment or serve as a standard of medical care. Variations, taking into
account individual circumstances, may be appropriate.

Introduction

The American Academy of Pediatrics (AAP) Task Force on Pediatric AIDS, established in 1987, was immediately faced with a number of controversial issues in the care and treatment of pediatric patients with HIV infection — school and day care attendance, foster care, appropriate infection control measures, and transmission of the virus. In 1987, diagnosis of HIV infection in the newborn was still a difficult problem. Many infants at risk for infection were identified only after they developed severe disease; voluntary testing and counseling for HIV infection were not widespread. The first policy statements published by the Task Force were instrumental in educating pediatricians and providing guidance for the care of HIV-infected children within the pediatric community. In 1992, the Task Force became the Provisional Committee on Pediatric AIDS and has been active in updating/revising prior statements and keeping the AAP membership abreast of new issues.

Since the recognition of pediatric HIV infection in the early 1980s, the number of HIV-infected children has increased steadily each year, spreading from urban communities into rural areas. What was once considered an acute illness with a high mortality has now evolved into a chronic, multisystem disease that has became one of the leading causes of death in infants, children, and adolescents in the United States. As with other chronic illnesses, the pediatrician plays an important role in the care of these individuals.

The Compendium of AAP Guidelines on Pediatric HIV Infection is designed to assist the pediatrician in caring for the multiple medical and psychosocial needs of children in various settings with HIV infection. As our knowledge of HIV infection evolves, this compendium will be updated and expanded. We thank you for your understanding, advocacy, and caring for children and their families with HIV infection.

Gwendolyn B. Scott, MD

Gwendolyn B. Scott, MD
Chairperson
AAP Provisional Committee on Pediatric AIDS
August 1994

Table of Contents

OSHA: Materials to Assist the Pediatric Office in Implementing the Bloodborne Pathogen, Hazard Communication, and Other OSHA Standards

Report of the Committee on Infectious Diseases

School Health: Policy and Practice

AAP Policy Statements

For information on ordering reprints
of AAP policy statements, contact:
American Academy of Pediatrics
Division of Publications
141 Northwest Point Blvd, PO Box 927
Elk Grove Village, IL 60009-0927
800/433-9016

AMERICAN ACADEMY OF PEDIATRICS

Committee on School Health

Acquired Immunodeficiency Syndrome Education in Schools (RE8123)

Aids Education

The AIDS epidemic has been with us for the past 6 years. As of October, 1987, 42,000 total cases of AIDS in persons of all ages have been reported, and the number is predicted to increase to 250,000 cases by 1991. Because no vaccine or cure is available, education offers a reasonable approach to prevention. The American Academy of Pediatrics believes that the nation's schools should immediately initiate AIDS education programs as part of a comprehensive health education plan.

ORGANIZATION OF THE PROGRAM

School Health Advisory Committee

AIDS education programs in the schools should be advocated for and supervised by a school health advisory committee or similar school-related organization in each community.[1] The committee for each school or district should consist of the school medical advisor, a community pediatrician and/or public health physician, a school nurse, a health educator, a mental health professional, a school administrator, and a faculty member, a parent, and appropriate community representatives. In smaller school systems, a single school health advisory committee should suffice. These programs should be coordinated by the school medical advisor, school administrators, and school nursing supervisor.

Physician and Nurse Training

Physicians, especially pediatricians and family physicians, and school nurses should receive train-

This statement has been approved by the Council on Child and Adolescent Health.

The recommendations in this statement do not indicate an exclusive course of treatment or procedure to be followed. Variations, taking into account individual circumstances, may be appropriate.

Reaffirmed 6/90

ing about AIDS by participating in educational programs sponsored by regional medical centers, state medical societies, state nursing organizations, public health departments, or organizations such as the state chapters of the American Academy of Pediatrics. Those trained would then: (1) conduct education programs for teachers, school administrators, parent groups, community groups, psychologists and other mental health personnel, and students; (2) assist schools and organizations in the development of educational programs for special groups; (3) review, adapt, and develop educational materials; (4) participate in public panel discussions, including radio and television programs; (5) take part in open discussions between school administrators and staff or between administrators and parents; and (6) facilitate networking among parents, educators, and AIDS support groups.

Educator Training

AIDS education in the schools should be taught in developmentally appropriate programs by qualified teachers. Ethnocultural differences among students must be considered carefully. At all levels, teachers should be experienced in child development and health, health education methods and materials, and the teaching of human sexuality.

Community Education

Parents and the community at large should be fully informed about the content of AIDS education programs in schools. They should also participate in curriculum development, evaluation, and revision with information updated at regular intervals.

CURRICULUM

Schools should provide a comprehensive program of health education in which health promotion and disease avoidance are emphasized. As part of this program, AIDS education should start in kindergarten and continue through 12th grade. From kindergarten to third grade, as a foundation, concepts of disease and health should be taught, including the role of microorganisms and the importance of cleanliness in maintaining a healthy body. The role of health professionals in preventing and treating illness in the family should be introduced.

In the fourth through sixth grades, the nature of AIDS and methods of transmission should be discussed, as well as concepts involving the control of body fluids. Myths about insect vectors and the casual spread of AIDS should be dispelled.

Schoolchildren in grades 7 through 12 begin to engage in behavior that may increase the risk of human immunodeficiency virus (HIV) infection. It is in this group, therefore, that the curriculum needs to be most intense. Although the regular classroom teacher can handle the early grades, professional health educators should be used in these later grades. Programs should consist of five topics: (1) the spectrum and natural history of AIDS as a sexually transmitted disease; (2) the relationship between the AIDS virus and the human immune system; (3) the transmission of the AIDS virus; (4) the prevention and treatment of AIDS; and (5) the social and psychologic aspects of AIDS.[2]

Students must understand how the AIDS virus is transmitted to understand its prevention. Candid discussion of all aspects of sexual transmission must occur in an age-appropriate and culturally sensitive fashion. Intravenous drug use with needle sharing should be emphasized as an important cause of AIDS transmission. In the past, blood products contaminated by virus caused disease. Present methods of screening and preparing blood have greatly reduced this problem. Congenital transmission from an infected mother to her baby is an important cause of AIDS.[3] Its prevention should be emphasized.

AIDS is a disease that has a complex social impact on children, families, schools, and the community. Curricula should emphasize an understanding of the psychologic problems of families with children or other members who have AIDS, a knowledge of alternate life-styles, special cultural sensitivities, civil rights, and testing issues.

PREVENTION

The prevention of AIDS can be incorporated into an overall approach to responsible sexual behavior and decision making that includes prevention of all sexually transmissible infections. The safest method of prevention is abstinence from sexual activity until one reaches psychosocial maturity and a mutually faithful relationship is established

with a person who never has been exposed to HIV. Because not all students will remain abstinent or be able to ensure that their sexual partners are uninfected, appropriate barrier methods should be discussed as part of the curriculum. The proper use of latex condoms and virucidal spermicides (contraceptive vaginal foams containing nonoxynol 9) should be described,[4] as well as the lack of protection against AIDS and other sexually transmitted diseases from use of oral contraceptives alone.

PROGRAM ASSESSMENT

AIDS education courses should be periodically evaluated by the school health advisory committee and regularly updated by the school medical advisor and public health experts to conform with current knowledge.

The American Academy of Pediatrics has been active in advocating health education in the schools[5] and the inclusion of children with AIDS into schools.[6] We now recommend that all physicians, especially pediatricians, supply leadership to help solve a growing AIDS crisis by encouraging the development of local AIDS education programs as we have done with family life education programs (*AAP News*, April 1986, p 14).

COMMITTEE ON SCHOOL HEALTH, 1987–1988
Martin C. Ushkow, MD, Chairman
Beverley J. Bayes, MD
Philip R. Nader, MD
Jerry Newton, MD
Steven R. Poole, MD
Martin W. Sklaire, MD

Liaison Representatives
Jeffrey L. Black, MD, American
   School Health Association
Patricia Lachelt, National Association of
   Pediatric Nurse Associates and Practitioners
Nick Staresinic, PhD, American Association of
   School Administrators
Bonnie Wilford, PhD, American Medical
   Association
Charles Zimont, MD, American Academy of
   Family Physicians

Consultant
Joseph Zanga, MD

REFERENCES

1. American Academy of Pediatrics, Committee on School Health: *School Health: A Guide for Health Professionals.* Elk Grove Village, IL, American Academy of Pediatrics, 1987, pp 15–16
2. *Acquired Immunodeficiency Syndrome (AIDS Secondary*

Level Curriculum Resources Packet). Hartford, CT, Connecticut Departments of Education and Health Services, April 1987

3. Recommendations for assisting in the prevention of perinatal transmission of human T-lymphotropic virus type III/lymphadenopathy-associated virus and acquired immunodeficiency syndrome. *MMWR* 1985;34:721–725, 731–732

4. Centers for Disease Control: Condoms for prevention of sexually transmitted diseases. *JAMA* 1988;259:1925–1927

5. American Academy of Pediatrics, Committee on School Health: Health education and schools. *Pediatrics* 1985; 75:1160–1161

6. American Academy of Pediatrics, Committees on School Health and Infectious Diseases: School attendance of children and adolescents with human T lymphotropic virus III/lymphadenopathy-associated virus infection. *Pediatrics* 1986;77:430–432

Useful AIDS Education Resource Materials for Teachers, Physicians and Nurses

1. *Acquired Immunodeficiency Syndrome (AIDS Secondary Level Curriculum Resources Packet)*. Hartford, Connecticut Departments of Education and Health Services, April 1987

2. *AIDS and Adolescents*. Resources for Educators, Education Department-Center for Population Options, 1012 14th St, NW Washington, DC 20005, July 1987

3. *AIDS Information/Education Plan to Prevent and Control AIDS in the United States*. US Department of Health and Human Services, Public Health Services, March 1987

4. *AIDS Instructional Guide for Teachers Grades K–12*. C/O Deputy Commissioner for Elementary, Secondary, and Continuing Education, State Education Department, University of New York, Albany, NY 12234, 1987

5. *Family Living Including Sex Education: Supplementary Material Related to AIDS*. New York City Board of Education, Office of Curriculum Development and Support, Office of the Chancellor, 110 Livingston St, Brooklyn, NY 11201, 1986

6. Centers for Disease Control: Guidelines for effective school health education to prevent the spread of AIDS. *MMWR* 1988;37:52

7. *Report of the Surgeon General's Workshop on Children with HIV Infection and Their Families: Recommendations of Work Group IV*. US Department of Health and Human Services, Public Health Service, DHHS publication No. HRS-D-MC87-1, April 1987

8. *SIECUS Report*, vol XV, No. VII. Sex Information and Education Council of the US Inc, New York University, 32 Washington Place, New York, NY 10003, July–August 1987, pp 1–5, 11–17

9. *Teacher Curriculum Guide on AIDS*. C/O Elizabeth Stoller, Department of Public Health, Bureau of Disease Control, 101 Grove St, San Francisco, CA 94102, 1987

AMERICAN ACADEMY OF PEDIATRICS

Addressing Concerns of Pediatric Trainees Caring for Patients With Human Immunodeficiency Virus Infection (RE9330)

Task Force on Pediatric AIDS

Since the recognition of the human immunodeficiency virus (HIV) as the cause of HIV infection and the acquired immunodeficiency syndrome (AIDS), studies have determined that the risk of infection to the health care worker through occupational exposure is extremely low.[1-3] However, the perception of risk can have potential psychologic consequences for health care workers providing medical care to HIV-infected patients.[4] What is it that makes caring for HIV-infected patients an unsettling emotional experience? While occupational risks accompany all work, physicians have in the recent past perceived themselves with little vulnerability to a devastating disease.[5,6] Medical professionals at the turn of the century had alarmingly high rates of mortality from tuberculosis, and today, if not immunized, they are at increased risk for hepatitis B. HIV infection carries formidable biologic and social consequences that contribute to the psychologic stress that may accompany caring for infected patients.

Because HIV-infected patients are dealt with extensively in tertiary centers, there are significant implications for resident and medical student training, especially in urban locales where the rate of HIV infection is high.[7-12]

The emotional risks of caring for patients with HIV infection have had scant documentation, but there is growing evidence for concern. A study of 250 residents in New York City documented that 19% of pediatric residents and 36% of medical residents had needle-stick exposure to HIV in 1986.[13] A 1988 study of 294 pediatric residents in 11 New York City programs revealed that 205 of the residents (69.7%) had been stuck with a blood-contaminated needle on 588 separate occasions.[14] While there was considerable concern expressed by residents over acquiring HIV, more than half did not want to know whether they were HIV seropositive. Only 11 of the 48 residents with needle-stick injuries of potentially HIV-contaminated blood received counseling or HIV testing after exposure.[13] Similar studies have not been reported in low-incidence locales.

The consequences of such exposures are sobering; 25% of New York City residents declared that if given a choice they would not care for AIDS patients; 53% of internal medicine and 44% of pediatric residents said they were resentful of having to take care of AIDS patients.[13]

In addition to the apprehension that accompanies the risk of accidental exposure, there are other aspects of dealing with patients with AIDS that can be disturbing to physicians in training. These include the following: (1) AIDS patients often die, placing stress on the health care professional in coping with loss and perceived failure; (2) patients or infected parents are usually young, often the same age as the resident, and this may cause anxiety because of physician identification with the patients; (3) adolescents and children with HIV infection and their families often have social problems that can foster a sense of anger, frustration, and futility. These feelings can be aggravated by stress and fatigue, common factors during residency training. Again, it should be noted that many of these kinds of reactions are not unique to HIV infections. Residents are often devastated by the death of patients, particularly young patients, regardless of cause. Further frustration in dealing with the overwhelming problems of inner-city populations is common.

Reports of the Presidential Commission on the HIV Epidemic[15] and the Institute of Medicine of the National Academy of Sciences[16] recommend dissemination of information about risks and risk-reduction techniques to health care providers. These have been codified by the 1992 Occupational Safety and Health Administration regulations.

The Association of American Medical Colleges (AAMC) has released a policy statement addressing the responsibilities of institutions toward trainees concerning HIV infection as well as policies for dealing with HIV-infected trainees.[17] The AAMC Guidelines include the following recommendations:

Institutions should develop and regularly review policies for dealing with HIV infections and possible exposure in health care staff. Institutions should devise policies to promote safe and appropriate patient care, confidentiality for HIV-infected individuals, a safe environment, and implementation of current laws. Modification of training or privileges for HIV-infected providers should be determined on an individual basis. Policies also need to be developed for ensuring and providing compensation for trainees infected as a result of caring for patients.

The Academy supports these recommendations and recommends that all training programs develop

PEDIATRICS (ISSN 0031 4005). Copyright © 1993 by the American Academy of Pediatrics.

specific policies designed to help students and residents care for patients with HIV infection in a safe and effective manner. It is also important to establish policies with respect to medical students who are not institutional employees. Such policies should describe explicit measures for dealing with the emotional consequences of caring for patients with HIV infection and the emotional consequences of being placed at risk of contracting a fatal illness. Institutions should develop programs and policies that address specific local needs as well as addressing the following areas:

Education About HIV Exposure Risks. Training programs should disseminate accurate and current information concerning HIV infection. Residents and students should know the probability of acquiring HIV infection following needle-stick exposure and of appropriate avoidance techniques. Information should be updated frequently. Available written and audiovisual material should be reviewed periodically.

Information should also address the psychologic consequences of exposure. It is necessary but not sufficient to inform an exposed individual that, according to current data, the risk of acquiring HIV infection after needle-stick exposure is 0.4%. The individual exposed to HIV through a needle-stick may consider only two outcomes: infection will or will not occur. This may be felt as a 50/50 chance of acquiring a fatal disease. It is essential to appreciate this phenomenon in order to address seriously the resident's concern. Therefore, we recommend a dual approach: address the facts and acknowledge the feelings that accompany the facts.

Expectations to Provide Care to HIV-Infected Patients. Training institutions have accepted the responsibility of caring for HIV-infected patients. Therefore, residents are obligated to care for assigned patients. Although not institutional employees, medical students are also expected to have clinical involvement with a variety of conditions, including HIV infection. It should be explicitly stated to residents and students that they will participate in the care of patients with HIV infection. Occasionally, a resident has refused to provide care for patients with AIDS. A formal written policy detailing the way in which the training program will respond to a resident's refusal should be in place.

Trainees should be assigned to clinical experiences commensurate with their ability and experience. They should be taught to perform procedures competently and safely as well as to cope emotionally with the risks that accompany those procedures. When requested and appropriate, medical students should also be expected to do venipunctures and assist in surgical procedures after they have received specific education and training and have suitable experience. Institutions should establish policies and promote safety during routine drawing of blood from known HIV-positive and other high-risk patients. Accidents increase when individuals are tired, and residents working long shifts are subject to fatigue.

Institutions should also develop explicit policies regarding the care of HIV-infected patients by pregnant students and residents. Pregnancy is currently not known to increase the risk of acquiring HIV infection after accidental exposure. Therefore, the biologic risk to the pregnant and nonpregnant resident is the same. Pregnant trainees may express apprehension that HIV acquired in a medical accident will infect their fetus as well. Based on current estimates of HIV seroconversion of 0.4% following needle-stick injury with HIV-seropositive blood and an estimated 33% likelihood of an infant of an HIV-infected mother acquiring HIV, there will be approximately 1 infected fetus per 750 needle-stick injuries with HIV-infected blood. The likelihood of accidental injury and exposure to infectious material can be reduced with adherence to proper techniques. The Academy recommends pregnant and nonpregnant trainees should have the same responsibilities in caring for HIV-infected patients.

Clear policies should also exist as to expectations of all hospital personnel caring for HIV-infected patients. There have been reports of other hospital personnel refusing to participate in the care of patients with HIV. In these situations, some residents have felt both obligated to provide care and victimized by having to accept responsibility to give the care that other hospital personnel have refused to provide. Care for HIV-infected patients is an obligation of all hospital personnel. Trainees should not be required to assume the responsibilities that others have avoided.

Minimizing Risk in Patient Care Settings. Universal precautions are mandated for dealing with blood and blood products in health care institutions.[19] One of the major reasons for the lack of appropriate use of precautions has been the lack of availability and accessibility of appropriate material in areas where resuscitations and other expedient procedures are conducted. In addition, it is essential that materials of the highest quality be available and that varying sizes be provided. A common reason given for not using gloves in appropriate situations, cited especially by female residents, is that only one size is available and that size is too large to accomplish a technical procedure comfortably and accurately.

Residents working in emergency departments must be especially cognizant of risks of needle-stick injuries. Needles and syringes used for emergency procedures such as intracardiac injections have been laid on or stuck into examining tables or dropped on the floor during emergencies. The risk of needle-stick for other hospital personnel is particularly high in these situations.

It is also essential to monitor whether or not precautions are being followed. This monitoring should be done routinely and regularly. If precautions are not followed, it is important to meet with housestaff to discuss and remove barriers to implementation.

Formal Departmental Mechanisms for Dealing With Concerns About HIV Infections. Each department should have identified resource personnel who can address the medical and psychologic concerns of housestaff about AIDS. There should be regularly scheduled meetings in which issues of exposure risk and the emotional aspects of caring for patients with HIV infection are openly discussed.

Housestaff and students should also have access to information or counseling sessions in an environment of complete confidentiality. Counseling should be available from individuals who do not have influence over a trainee's status in a residency program. At the request of any student or resident, confidential HIV testing should be available, with appropriate and confidential counseling both before and after testing. To guarantee confidentiality, trainees should be advised of the availability of anonymous testing sites. Institutions should provide initial and follow-up testing at no charge to individuals who experience either needle-stick or splash exposures.

Each department should have in place a protocol for dealing with exposure to blood and blood-contaminated body fluid from patients with known or unknown HIV status. In high-risk areas, 24-hour availability of individuals who are on call and competent in current medical and psychologic approaches to management of accidental injury is recommended. The efficacy of zidovudine taken prophylactically following needle-stick injury has not been proven to be of benefit, but the risks and potential benefits of such therapy should be discussed with a resident who has had an accidental stick.[18] Hepatitis B immunoglobulin should be considered if the resident has not been immunized against hepatitis B.

In addition, each department should have a mandatory session for general counseling and information purposes. Needle-stick injury with HIV-infected blood has on occasion caused psychologic distress of such magnitude as to warrant disability leave. Health professionals often resist seeking appropriate mental health care. The greatest difficulty is making the initial encounter. A mandatory group meeting would provide a nonstigmatizing means of making an initial contact. After needle-stick or other high-risk exposure, individual counseling sessions should be strongly encouraged. Institutions in high-risk areas should be aware of the need for such services, and insurance should cover the cost of counseling in order to promote adjustment after exposure.

Institutions should deal with issues such as (1) the support and acceptance of residents with HIV infection into the training program and continuation of the training of residents who themselves have HIV infection; (2) the educational balance in training programs with a large number of HIV-infected patients; and (3) the economic, medical, and social consequences for trainees who acquire HIV at work. The report by the AAMC outlines many of these issues, and this report is suggested as a guide for policy development by individual programs and institutions.[17]

ACADEMY RECOMMENDATIONS

1. All pediatric trainees should be expected to care for patients with HIV infection.
2. Residents and medical students should be knowledgeable about the modes of transmission and methods of prevention of HIV infection. Institutions should establish policies, promote infection-control safeguards, and monitor adherence to safety policies and universal precautions.
3. Training programs should address the emotional aspects of caring for patients with HIV infection as part of their formal curriculum.
4. Institutions should have policies for dealing with the medical, psychosocial, and economic consequences of HIV exposure by residents and medical students.
5. Confidential HIV testing should be available on request, without charge, and should be accompanied by pretest and posttest counseling. Counseling given before the testing should include discussion of the impact of HIV status on career development in accordance with evolving guidelines and recommendations. Trainees should be made aware of the availability of anonymous testing sites.

TASK FORCE ON PEDIATRIC AIDS, 1991 to 1992
Stanley A. Plotkin, MD, Chairperson
Louis Z. Cooper, MD
Hugh E. Evans, MD
Norman C. Fost, MD, MPH
Sherrel L. Hammar, MD
Alfred Healy, MD
Renee Jenkins, MD
Gerald Merenstein, MD
Robert H. Pantell, MD
S. Kenneth Schonberg, MD
Gwendolyn B. Scott, MD
Martin W. Sklaire, MD

Liaison Representative
Martha F. Rogers, MD, Centers for Disease Control

Consultant
James R. Allen, MD, MPH, National AIDS Program Office

AAP Staff
Edgar O. Ledbetter, MD, Director, Department of Maternal, Child & Adolescent Health

REFERENCES

1. Henerson DK, Fahey BJ, Willy M, et al. Risk for occupational transmission of human immunodeficiency virus type 1 (HIV-1) associated with clinical exposures: a prospective evaluation. *Ann Intern Med.* 1990;113:740–746
2. Marcus R. CDC Cooperative Needlestick Study Group. Surveillance of health-care workers exposed to blood from patients infected with the human immunodeficiency virus. *N Engl J Med.* 1988;319:1118–1123
3. Centers for Disease Control. Update: human immunodeficiency virus infections in health-care workers exposed to blood of infected patients. *MMWR.* 1987;36:285–289
4. Treiber FA, Shaw D, Malcolm R. Acquired immune deficiency syndrome: psychological impact on health personnel. *J Nerv Ment Dis.* 1987;175:496–499
5. Annas GJ. Not saints, but healers: the legal duties of health care professionals in the AIDS epidemic. *Am J Public Health.* 1988;78:844–849
6. Brandt AM. AIDS in historical perspective: four lessons from the history of sexually transmitted diseases. *Am J Public Health.* 1988;78:367–371
7. Brennan TA. The acquired immunodeficiency syndrome (AIDS) as an occupational disease. *Ann Intern Med.* 1987;107:581–583
8. Cooke M. Housestaff attitudes toward the acquired immunodeficiency syndrome. *AIDS Public Policy J.* 1988;3:59–60
9. Cooke M, Sande MA. The HIV epidemic training in internal medicine: challenges and recommendations. *N Engl J Med.* 1989;321:1334–1338
10. Imperato PJ, Feldman JG, Nayer K, DeHovitz JA. Medical students'

attitudes towards caring for patients with AIDS in a high incidence area. *NY State J Med.* 1988;88:223–227

11. Wachter RM. The impact of the acquired immunodeficiency syndrome on medical residency training. *N Engl J Med.* 1986;314:177–180

12. Whalen JP. Participation of medical students in the care of patients with AIDS. *J Med Educ.* 1987;62:53–54

13. Link RN, Feingold AR, Charap MH, Freeman K, Shelov SP. Concerns of medical and pediatric house officers about acquiring AIDS from their patients. *Am J Public Health.* 1988;78:455–459

14. Melzer S, Vermund SH, Shelov SP. Needlestick injuries among pediatric house officers in New York City. *AJDC.* 1989;143:430

15. Presidential Commission. *Report of the Presidential Commission on the Human Immunodeficiency Virus Epidemic: June 24, 1988.* Washington, DC: US Government Printing Office; 1988

16. Institute of Medicine, National Academy of Sciences. *Confronting AIDS: Update 1988.* Washington, DC: National Academy Press; 1988

17. Association of American Medical Colleges. Policy Guidelines for Addressing HIV Infection in the Academic Medical Community: A Report of the AAMC Committee on AIDS and the Academic Medical Center. Washington, DC: Association of Medical Colleges; October 1988

18. US Dept of Health Human Services, Public Health Service. Public Health Service statement on management of occupational exposure to human immunodeficiency virus, including considerations regarding zidovudine postexposure use. *MMWR.* 1990;39:1–14

19. US Dept of Health Human Services, Public Health Service. Recommendations for preventing transmission of human immunodeficiency virus and hepatitis B virus to patients during exposure-prone invasive procedures. *MMWR.* 1991;40:1–9

AMERICAN ACADEMY OF PEDIATRICS

Adolescents and Human Immunodeficiency Virus Infection: The Role of the Pediatrician in Prevention and Intervention (RE9331)

Task Force on Pediatric AIDS

The incidence of human immunodeficiency virus (HIV) infection among adolescents is both significant and rising, and concern about this disease is increasingly evident among adolescents, their parents, and health professionals. Such concern evolves from multiple factors including not only the number of adolescents who have been reported to have the acquired immunodeficiency syndrome (AIDS), but also the uncertainty as to how many youths have been infected with the virus but remain asymptomatic; the risk of becoming infected through either heterosexual behavior, homosexual behavior, or substance abuse; and the need to implement effective preventive strategies.

EPIDEMIOLOGY

By the end of December 1992, a total of 946 cases of AIDS in persons aged 13 through 19 had been reported to the Centers for Disease Control. Although adolescents account for less than 1% of the total reported cases of AIDS, 20% of total cases occur in young adults aged 20 through 29.[1]

The long latency period between infection with HIV and the emergence of clinical AIDS, often in excess of 5 years, suggests that many of these young adults were first infected during their adolescence. For others, who become infected as young adults, the sexual or drug use behaviors that placed them at risk for infection had their onset during adolescence.

Although national cross-sectional seroprevalence studies have not been conducted, data from selected populations of adolescents provide some information about the rate of infection among segments of the adolescent population. Since October 1985, the Department of Defense has tested applicants for military service for HIV infection. The prevalence rate for 17- to 19-year-olds screened between October 1985 and March 1989 was 0.34 per 1000.[2] The rate was more than 10-fold higher among nearly 70 000 Job Corps applicants screened between October 1987 and November 1988, with 3.9 per 1000 being infected. Among nearly 14 000 students using health services at 17 college campuses, the seroprevalence rate was 1.7 per 1000,[3] while at another extreme, the rate among homeless youth seen at a shelter in New York City was 88 per 1000.[4] Although these data cannot be reliably generalized to the entire adolescent population, they do provide insight into the extent of the problem among adolescents and young adults.

To date, for those who have manifested AIDS during their adolescence, males have outnumbered females in a ratio of 4:1, compared to an adult male-female ratio of 9:1. The receipt of blood or blood products prior to 1985 accounts for nearly 40% of all cases of AIDS in adolescents. Hemophilia and other coagulation disorders are associated with approximately three fourths of these cases, which occur predominantly in males. However, as a result of the success of current methods of testing donated blood for the presence of HIV, this risk factor represents a decreasing proportion of young people with AIDS. Homosexual and bisexual contact in males, representing one fourth of cases among 13- through 19-year-olds, is the next most frequent risk behavior, followed by heterosexual contact in males and females (approximately 14%) and injection drug abuse (approximately 13%). Among adolescent females, heterosexual contact is the most frequent risk factor (approximately 45%), followed by injection drug abuse (approximately 27%). Female sexual partners of high-risk males comprise approximately 12% of all adolescents with AIDS, representing a significantly higher proportion of cases secondary to heterosexual transmission than has been reported for adults (approximately 2.5%). Male and female prostitution, especially among homeless and runaway youth, should be acknowledged as a factor increasing the risk of HIV acquisition.

Both the increased proportion of adolescent females with AIDS secondary to heterosexual transmission and the lower male-female ratio encountered in adolescents ($\approx$4:1 vs $\approx$9:1 in adults) remain, in part, unexplained. These differences may be secondary to the fact that the initial wave of this epidemic impacted most heavily on adult homosexual males and that the current trend of the epidemic, which now includes adolescents, evidences a more equal distribution among the sexes. That adolescent girls are more likely to have older sex partners, who are hence more likely to be infected, also places them at increased risk. In addition, there is an association between adolescent crack/cocaine abuse and the risk of acquiring HIV infection. This risk almost certainly relates to sexual practices involved in obtaining drugs or money for drugs.[5]

These data demonstrate that behaviors common to adolescents, including emerging sexuality, substance abuse, running away, and homelessness, may place them at risk for HIV infection. Preventing such in-

PEDIATRICS (ISSN 0031 4005). Copyright © 1993 by the American Academy of Pediatrics.

fection and addressing the concerns of those young people who may already be infected has become a part of adolescent health care.

COUNSELING THE ADOLESCENT

Information regarding sexually transmitted diseases, including HIV infection and AIDS, should be included as an important component of the anticipatory guidance provided by pediatricians to their adolescent patients.[6] The majority of young people will have had a first sexual intercourse experience either during their adolescent years or as young adults. The risk of exposure to HIV for a particular adolescent will vary with geographic location, sexual practices, and other high-risk behaviors. However, there is no way that a person can be certain that a potential sexual partner is not infected with HIV because of prior sexual experiences, injection drug abuse, or blood transfusion. Hence there is never certainty that a partner is free from HIV infection.

Every adolescent contemplating or engaging in sexual intercourse will need to be concerned and knowledgeable about HIV infection. This new threat of exposure to a fatal sexually transmitted disease adds to the necessity of discussing sexuality with adolescent patients. Abstinence from sexual intercourse is the safest course of action. Alternatives to sexual intercourse should be discussed with the adolescent contemplating or engaged in sexual behavior. Many adolescents will not refrain from sexual intercourse. It is very difficult to predict which adolescents will or will not remain abstinent, and, therefore, safer sex practices including condom use should be addressed with these young people.[6,7]

Addressing the consequences of drug abuse has become a mandatory part of the health care of adolescents. Drug abuse is common and carries a significant risk of transmission of HIV through needle-sharing practices. A young person engaged in injection drug abuse is unlikely to forgo that experience because of the fear of HIV infection, but the pediatrician should nevertheless include AIDS on the list of risks inherent to such behavior.

Such counseling on issues of sexuality, drug abuse, and risk reduction may be more effective when done by those of similar race, social class, gender, or age of the patient, utilizing community resources where possible.[8]

COUNSELING ADOLESCENTS AT HIGH RISK

Some adolescents are at particularly high risk of contracting HIV infection, because of either behaviors or circumstances that increase the likelihood that they have been or will be exposed to the virus. These include drug abusers; homosexual and bisexual youth, including both male and female prostitutes; and adolescents with a history of sexually transmitted diseases, in particular herpes or syphilis[9–11]; adolescents with multiple sexual partners; and those whose sexual partners have engaged in high-risk behaviors. Also at risk of having contracted HIV infection are young people who have a history of transfusion of blood or blood products prior to April 1985. General advice would be applicable to all adolescents at high risk, while other recommendations would be specific to the behavior or condition that places the young person at risk.

All adolescents at high risk should be given the most recent information about AIDS, including etiology, routes of transmission, and the consequences of HIV infection. Discussion will also need to address the availability and implications of testing for the presence of HIV, the current status of our knowledge regarding the course and treatment of this disease, measures they can use to protect themselves from acquiring this infection, and the reality that if they are infected they are capable of transmitting this disease to others including their sex partners and their offspring.

The issues surrounding testing for HIV infection need to focus on the advantages and disadvantages of determining an adolescent's serostatus. Among the advantages of such a determination would be that a negative HIV test result can reduce the anxiety associated with risk status (it should be recognized, however, that antibodies may not appear for several months following infection). For many, a positive result will be better than not knowing. Knowing a positive result will facilitate reasoned planning of future behavior that affects not only the welfare of the adolescent but also the potential for spreading the disease. In addition, new advances in the treatment of AIDS such as antiretroviral drugs and pneumocystis prophylaxis offer benefit to the infected person. The discussion of drawbacks should include the psychological stress that most individuals encounter in dealing with knowing that they are infected with HIV and the almost certain need for additional counseling in such cases. In addition, the adolescent must be told that although efforts will be made to protect confidentiality, it cannot be guaranteed, and that a young person who is known to be HIV seropositive may very well face social, educational, economic, and vocational consequences. These problems, which might diminish the willingness of an adolescent to seek testing, should be balanced by the potential benefits of knowing one's HIV status.

All high-risk adolescents and those who either have AIDS or are known to be HIV seropositive should be made aware that they can transmit this potentially fatal infection to others. Even those at high risk but with a negative test for HIV may in the future show evidence of the virus, particularly if they continue to engage in the high-risk behavior, and at that point they would be capable of spreading the disease. Counsel should include emphasis on the adolescent's obligation to protect others and to inform sexual partners who are being or who may already have been exposed. The protection of others would include abstinence from sexual intercourse or the use of safer sex practices, including the proper use of condoms. HIV-seropositive adolescents may exhibit either reluctance or refusal to inform their sexual partners of their serostatus. In such cases the pediatrician should offer assistance in informing the sexual partner or offer the assistance of public health officials expert in contact tracing. In some cases, when faced with persistent refusal, the pediatrician may have an obligation to disclose over the objections of the patient (see "Consent and Confidentiality" section below).

Other aspects of counseling would be directed to the behavior that places the adolescent at risk. The AIDS epidemic provides additional import and poignancy to the need for drug abusers to be offered treatment for their addiction, and young people who might otherwise refuse therapeutic intervention may now accept such advice because of a fear of HIV infection. Discussion of the dangers of sharing needles and methods for sterilizing needles may be appropriate for the adolescent who continues injection drug abuse despite all efforts to interrupt this behavior. Sexually active adolescents should be informed of the risk of continued exposure so they might opt to alter their sexual behavior by abstaining from sexual intercourse, or sustaining monogamous relationships, and using condoms and engaging in "safer sex." Adolescents at risk because of prior treatment with blood products should understand that heat treatment of factor VIII and HIV testing of such blood products has greatly reduced the risk from transfusions given after April 1985.

Adolescents with a sexually transmitted disease, in particular herpes or syphilis, should be informed about the association between these conditions and the transmission of HIV. Although the basis for this association is unclear, and may relate to either the behaviors that led to the sexually transmitted disease (promiscuity, prostitution, intimacy with a high-risk partner) or genital lesions predisposing to the transmission of HIV, the adolescent should be counseled about behavioral changes that would minimize future risk of HIV and other sexually transmitted diseases.

Some adolescents will have sexual partners who are either known to be HIV seropositive or who have engaged in high-risk behaviors. The counseling alternatives in such circumstances would include suggesting termination of the relationship or minimizing risk through practicing "safer sex." At the least, these young people need be made aware of the risk of sexual transmission of HIV infection and how to avoid infection. Female adolescents should be made aware of the risks of transmission of HIV to their offspring and the consequences of perinatal infection.

CONSENT AND CONFIDENTIALITY

Adults (in general, individuals 18 years of age or older) may consent to their own medical care. Similarly, emancipated minors (individuals younger than the age of 18 but self-supporting, married, parents themselves, or members of the armed services) may consent to their own health care without the need for parental involvement. In addition, public health statutes and legal precedents allow for the medical evaluation and treatment of minors for certain categorical illnesses, in particular sexually transmitted diseases, without parental knowledge or consent. To date, however, HIV infection has not been clearly defined as a condition for which evaluation or treatment of a minor may proceed without parental consent.

At times, an adolescent may not wish to involve a parent in decisions relative to either evaluation or treatment for HIV infection. Such reluctance may arise from a desire not to inform family members about HIV status or not to reveal the behaviors that placed the adolescent at risk for infection including substance abuse and homosexual or heterosexual activity. Although it is often best to involve the family in the health care of the adolescent, such is not always the case. Deference to parental opinion or parental wishes to be informed should not interfere with needed evaluation or treatment of the adolescent.[12] For the adolescent who is able to understand the implications of testing and treatment, and hence capable of informed consent, in the absence of local laws to the contrary, it would be best to proceed on the basis of this consent alone, rather than insisting on parental involvement. Similarly, the consent of the capable adolescent should be obtained prior to the release of any information concerning HIV status.

Individuals with HIV infection or AIDS, and their family members, have been the subject of educational, economic, and vocational discrimination, social ostracism, and even physical violence. In addition, since the disease can be transmitted through sexual intercourse, the individual identified as having HIV infection may lose his or her sexual partner and/or have difficulty finding new ones. Because of the psychosocial and socioeconomic implications of this disease, it is understandable that many at risk would opt to avoid HIV testing, or if tested, would request strict confidentiality regarding all aspects of their condition.

Questions about whether a pediatrician should disclose or receive information about a patient's HIV status without the consent of the patient may arise in several contexts including disclosure by obstetricians to pediatricians, mandated reporting to health departments, reporting to institutional authorities and employers, the care of accused or convicted sex offenders, instances of accidental needle-sticks involving known HIV seropositive patients, and issues of charting HIV status. Although each of these contexts may at times involve an adolescent patient, they are not specific to young people and are beyond the scope of this paper. A concern most relevant to the care of HIV-seropositive adolescents is the limits of confidentiality as they would apply to sexual partners.

A difficult question is whether to disclose HIV status to the sexual partner of a patient who is known to be HIV seropositive and who persistently refuses to agree to such disclosure. There should be little debate about the desirability of using all reasonable means to persuade an infected patient to inform his or her partner on a voluntary basis. Debate arises primarily over the patient who persistently refuses to inform or to allow others to inform his or her partner, for the understandable reason that the relationship may be terminated, as well as because of fears of wider disclosure.

In the context of whether or not to inform sexual partners, there has been considerable discussion of the "Tarasoff" rule—a legal principle that requires psychotherapists in some states to report patients who intend to kill an identifiable third person—and its relevance to disclosure of HIV infection.[13] The Tarasoff cases are not analogous to patients with HIV infection for two reasons. The former involve clearly criminal behavior—the intentional killing of another person. In addition, the victims in the Tarasoff cases have no way of protecting themselves. While potential victims of HIV infection may be unaware of their partner's HIV status, most can protect themselves by taking precautions that have been widely promulgated, and recommended for all sexual relations, particularly when the HIV status of the partner is unknown. Certainly, the physician's duty to disclose will be higher when he or she is also the physician for the unsuspecting partner. There is also a stronger argument for disclosure when the relationship is a stable one, in which the partner has little reason to suspect that his or her mate is at risk for HIV infection. When a physician believes there is a duty to disclose a patient's HIV status to the patient's sexual partner without the consent of the patient, it would be preferable to use the health department for such notification. Health departments are more likely to have the time and experience in contact tracing and notification, as well as familiarity with relevant law.

Whether a physician has an ethical duty to a patient depends on several factors, particularly the following:

- Whether he or she has contracted (promised) to care for that person
- Whether there are laws that create such a duty
- Whether commonly accepted codes of ethics identify such a duty

The only clear legal duty in the clinical setting of HIV infection is to the primary patient. The situation will be more complicated if the unsuspecting sexual partner is also a patient of the same physician. Absent that, the duty to a third party is unclear, in contrast to the clear duty to the primary patient.

In summary, several factors should be considered in deciding whether to disclose a patient's HIV status to a sexual partner without the consent of the patient:

A. Whether the physician has an established relationship or other preexisting duty to the partner at risk.
B. Whether the partner has reasonable cause to suspect the risk or take precautions even without specific warning.
C. The likelihood that the partner is, in fact, at risk. If, for example, appropriate precautions are being used, the risk of transmission may be low.
D. Relevant law, which may prohibit or require such disclosures. Principles of confidentiality may preclude such disclosures, whereas the possibility of a suit for negligence may require it.
E. Possible effects on future patients, either of the particular physician or patients in general. The realization that physicians will disclose such in-

formation without consent will presumably deter many individuals from seeking HIV testing or counseling.

Physicians who intend to disclose to patients' sexual partners should consider their duty to inform their patients prior to testing that test results will be disclosed to partners, and under what circumstances.

CONCLUSIONS AND RECOMMENDATIONS

1. Information regarding HIV infection and AIDS should be regarded as an important component of the anticipatory guidance provided by pediatricians to their adolescent patients. This guidance should include information about transmission, implications of infection, and strategies for prevention including abstinence from behaviors that place adolescents at risk and safer sex practices for those who opt to be sexually active.
2. Young people at risk for HIV infection should be offered diagnostic testing in addition to other educational and counseling services.
3. Parental involvement in adolescent health care is a desirable goal; however, the consent of the adolescent alone should be sufficient to provide evaluation and treatment for suspected or confirmed HIV infection.
4. The maintenance of confidentiality regarding HIV status is of great importance. Respecting this confidentiality, the pediatrician should use all reasonable means to persuade an infected adolescent to inform his or her sexual partner on a voluntary basis. Involuntary disclosure is a complex question that should be decided on the basis of local law, the relationship between the physician and the patient, the relationship of the physician to the patient's sexual partner, and the degree of perceived risk to the unsuspecting sexual partner.

TASK FORCE ON PEDIATRIC AIDS, 1991 to 1992
Stanley A. Plotkin, MD, Chairperson
Louis Z. Cooper, MD
Hugh E. Evans, MD
Norman C. Fost, MD, MPH
Sherrel L. Hammar, MD
Alfred Healy, MD
Renee Jenkins, MD
Gerald Merenstein, MD
Robert H. Pantell, MD
S. Kenneth Schonberg, MD
Gwendolyn B. Scott, MD
Martin W. Sklaire, MD

Liaison Representative
Martha F. Rogers, MD, Centers for Disease Control

Consultant
James R. Allen, MD, MPH, National AIDS Program Office

AAP Staff
Edgar O. Ledbetter, MD, Director, Department of Maternal, Child & Adolescent Health

REFERENCES

1. Centers for Disease Control and Prevention, National Center for Infectious Diseases, Division of HIV/AIDS. *HIV/AIDS Surveillance, Year End*

– 15 –

Edition. Cases Reported Through December 1992. Bethesda, MD: US Dept of Health and Human Services, US Public Health Service; 1992

2. Burke DS, Brundage JF, Goldenbaum M, et al. Human immunodeficiency virus in teenagers: seroprevalence among applicants for US military service. *JAMA.* 1990;263:2072–2077

3. Gayle HD, Keeling RP, Garcia-Tunon M, et al. Prevalence of the human immunodeficiency virus among university students. *N Engl J Med.* 1990;323:1538–1541

4. National Research Council. Miller HG, Turner CF, Moses LE, eds. *AIDS, The Second Decade.* Washington, DC: National Academy Press; 1990:152–159

5. Futterman DC, Hein K, Legg N, Dell R, Shaffer N. Comparison of HIV+ and HIV- high risk adolescents in a New York City HIV clinic. Presented at the VII International Conference on AIDS; June 1991; Florence, Italy

6. American Academy of Pediatrics, Committee on Adolescence. Contraception and adolescence. *Pediatrics.* 1990;86:134–138

7. American Academy of Pediatrics, Committee on School Health.

Acquired immune deficiency education in schools. *Pediatrics.* 1988;82:278–280

8. Slap GB, Plotkin SL, Khalid N, Michelman DF, Forke CM. A human immunodeficiency virus peer education program for adolescent females. *J Adolesc Health Care.* 1991;12:434–442

9. Stamm WE, Handsfield H, Rompalo AM, et al. The association between genital ulcer disease and acquisition of HIV infection in homosexual men. *JAMA.* 1988;260:1429–1433

10. Greenblatt RM, Lukehart SA, Plummer FA, et al. Genital ulceration as a risk factor for human immunodeficiency virus infection. *AIDS.* 1988;2:47–50

11. Wasserheit, JN. Epidemiological synergy: interrelationships between human immunodeficiency virus infection other sexually transmitted diseases. *Sex Transm Dis.* 1992;19:61–77

12. American Academy of Pediatrics. Confidentiality in adolescent health care. *AAP News.* April 1989

13. Gostin L, Curran WJ. AIDS screening, confidentiality and the duty to warn. *Am J Public Health.* 1987;77:361–365

AMERICAN ACADEMY OF PEDIATRICS
Task Force on Pediatric AIDS

Education of Children with Human Immunodeficiency Virus Infection (RE9222)

Children with human immunodeficiency virus (HIV) infection can participate in all activities in school to the extent that their health permits. The ability of the school to educate these children will depend on the severity of the disease. HIV infection has a wide clinical spectrum ranging from the asymptomatic child to the child with mild symptoms to the child with progressive acquired immunodeficiency syndrome (AIDS) who is deteriorating clinically. The child who is HIV-seropositive but is asymptomatic in appearance and activity is indistinguishable from the well child. The education of this child should not differ from the education of other children. The child who develops symptomatic HIV infection, however, may have evidence of central nervous system dysfunction resulting in decreased cognitive function and poor academic performance. Behavioral problems due to the chronic illness and increasing family disruption may interfere further with education. Issues of confidentiality may limit communication with the school. These problems pose challenges to school personnel and pediatricians attempting to optimally serve children with HIV infection.

Children with HIV infection should not be excluded from school for the protection of other children or personnel, nor should they be isolated within the school setting.[1] Exclusion of HIV-infected children from school to protect that child's health is not required in most instances, and such decisions should be made by the physician in consultation with the child's parent or care giver. (American Academy of Pediatrics. AIDS and Ethical Issues. Manuscript in preparation). Participation in school provides a sense of normality for the HIV-infected child and offers opportunities for socialization that are important to child development. School attendance also promotes a sense of belonging and reduces feelings of isolation and rejection.[2,3] The pediatrician, acting as the child's advocate, should be familiar with those neurologic and behavioral aspects of HIV infection that are associated with educational impairment and should provide counseling to the family and school while maintaining appropriate confidentiality.

HIV INFECTION AND DEVELOPMENTAL DELAY

Children with symptomatic HIV infection may develop severe developmental disability including intellectual impairment. This may be a direct result of central nervous system infection with HIV, but other factors, such as perinatal drug exposure, malnutrition, and repeated infection, also can contribute.[4] Recent studies have shown that 78% to 93% of children with symptomatic HIV infection show some developmental abnormality.[5] Four characteristic courses have been described[6]: (1) rapidly progressive central nervous system deterioration; (2) subacute, but steadily progressive central nervous system dysfunction; (3) a subacute course punctuated by periods of stability followed by deterioration[7]; (4) a static course. Symptoms vary from a mild developmental delay to progressive disease with acquired microcephaly, developmental regression, spasticity, and growth failure. Even children who maintain a static course frequently show cognitive defects with visual-spatial and perceptual dysfunction.[7,8]

As more children are born with this infection and survive for longer periods of time, there will be an increasing need for developmental assessments to plan educational programs. The Education for All Handicapped Children Act (Public Law 94-142) stated that all handicapped children aged 3 years and older are entitled to a free and appropriate education in the least restrictive environment. Infants and toddlers with HIV infection who have significant developmental delay or who are at risk for such delays are eligible for assistance under The Education For All Handicapped Children Amendments (Public Law 99-457) and may be eligible for

PEDIATRICS (ISSN 0031 4005). Copyright © 1991 by the American Academy of Pediatrics.

special services depending on state regulations. In some states, they may also be eligible for special services because they are at increased risk of developmental delay and potential learning problems. Thus, public school educational programs must be available for HIV-infected children from preschool through the school years. The pediatrician is responsible for initiating developmental testing and for referring children to appropriate early intervention and educational programs.[9]

The school medical advisor, as a member of the pupil evaluation team, should work with the child's pediatrician or other physician to help determine educational plans.[10] He or she can also help to plan educational programs for faculty, students, parents, the community, and the media about HIV infection and the educational needs of the HIV-infected child.[11]

HIV AS A CHRONIC DISEASE

The child with symptomatic HIV infection should be regarded as a chronically health-impaired child.[12] School personnel need to be oriented to the needs of the child with chronic disease. To benefit from education, children with HIV infection need to have health services available in their schools.[13] Children who are capable should be allowed to self-administer medication while in school.[14] Teachers, as well as nurses, should be trained in recognition and management of emergencies.[15] School personnel should also be trained in routine procedures for handling of all blood and blood-containing body fluids. Homebound teaching should also be readily available, and school attendance policies need to be flexible. Physical education programs suitable for the needs of the developmentally disabled or chronically ill child should be developed. Depending upon their capabilities, children with progressive disease may require home instruction, occupational and physical therapy, or mental health services.

HOME INSTRUCTION

Due to intercurrent illness, children with symptomatic HIV infection may be absent from school frequently and may require home instruction until their condition improves. As the illness progresses, the child may need to be kept at home. Educational programs, including home teaching, should be provided promptly under the guidelines of Public Law 94-142 through the school special education coordinator working with the school medical advisor or the child's physician. The child's physician, together with the school nurse, should facilitate the transition between school and home instruction. The need for home instruction should be reviewed within the context and guidelines of the American Academy of Pediatrics Policy Statement on Home Instruction.[16]

HEALTH-RELATED THERAPY

Children with symptomatic HIV infection may demonstrate visual-spatial and perceptual dysfunction. Neurologic findings, including poor fine motor coordination, clumsy rapid alternating movements, or abnormal gait[6,7] have been demonstrated in 75%. Such children need occupational and/or physical therapy and speech/language help under appropriate medical supervision.

BEHAVIORAL ASPECTS

As in other chronic illnesses, children with symptomatic HIV infection frequently exhibit behavioral symptoms, such as anxiety, depression, anger, and withdrawal, that can interfere with educational efforts. These behavioral problems may be due to the neurodevelopmental effects of the disease or to the problems associated with family disruption, community rejection, and the resulting parental isolation, guilt, and alienation. In middle school, there may be additional emotional problems associated with physical changes, such as weight loss, and declining cognitive function. The family should be given maximum support by school mental health personnel.

TERMINAL ILLNESS

As the disease takes a downward course, the child's capacity to be educated diminishes. The school can continue to serve an important need by assisting the family with counseling and emotional support and instructing classmates about the appropriate response to children with chronic and terminal illness.[17]

CONFIDENTIALITY

As long as the presence of AIDS or HIV infection stigmatizes the patient and his family, confidentiality will continue to be an important issue in which the need to safeguard the rights of the patient must be balanced by the school's request for information. The primary responsibility of the pediatrician is to serve the patient and the family. Because of the possible occurrence of fear and hysteria in the school, it is particularly important that disclosure of the child's HIV status to anyone in the school be done only with the informed consent of the parents and age-appropriate assent of the child. Some parents may be unwilling to agree to even limited disclosure. This should not prevent the child from attending school. School absenteeism and the child's cognitive deficits that result in learning disabilities may require the use of special services, but these usually can be obtained without revealing the diagnosis. School personnel should realize that there are children with HIV infection about whom no one will be aware because the child is asymptomatic or undiagnosed. A successful AIDS education program, however, will reassure teachers about the nature of the disease and create a more accepting environment so that the school staff can feel more comfortable with educating the HIV-infected child if the diagnosis should become known.

HIV-infected children may need medication administered during the school day. These medications should be given in the manner developed for all children who require medication while in school as described previously.[14] Because the nature of the medication which may identify a child as previously HIV-infected, only those who are involved immediately with the medication decisions in school need to be informed. In most circumstances, only the school medical advisor and school nurse will need such information. The decision for this limited disclosure should be made by the child's physician and the parents (AAP. AIDS and ethical issues. Manuscript in preparation).

The child with HIV infection also should be protected against other contagious diseases, such as measles and chicken pox. Vigorous enforcement of immunization requirements in all school settings will reduce but not eliminate the risk of such exposures. Therefore, methods for protecting HIV-infected children from these exposures should be developed which fit local circumstance and family wishes for confidentiality.

CONCLUSION

As the incidence of HIV infection in children increases, so will the school population of children with this disease. With the advent of new drug therapy, it is likely that these children will have a longer survival resulting in an increasing number of HIV-infected children entering school. An understanding of the effect of chronic illness and the recognition of neurodevelopmental problems in these children is essential to provide appropriate educational programs. The Academy recommends that:

1. All children with HIV infection should receive an appropriate education that is adapted to their evolving special needs. The spectrum of needs differs with the stage of the disease.
2. HIV infection should be treated like other chronic illnesses that require special education and other related services.
3. Continuity of education must be assured whether at school or at home.
4. Because of the stigmatization that still exists with this disease, it is essential that confidentiality be maintained by limiting disclosures and disclosing information only with the informed consent of the parents or legal guardians and age-appropriate assent of the student.

TASK FORCE ON PEDIATRIC AIDS, 1990 to 1991

Stanley A. Plotkin, MD
  Chairman
Louis Z. Cooper, MD
Hugh E. Evans, MD
Norman C. Fost, MD, MPH
Alfred Healy, MD
Renee Jenskins, MD

Gerald Merenstein, MD
Robert H. Pantell, MD
S. Kenneth Schonberg, MD
Gwendolyn B. Scott, MD
Martin W. Sklaire, MD
Esther H. Wender, MD

Consultant
James R. Allen, MD, MPH

REFERENCES

1. American Academy of Pediatrics, Task Force on Pediatric AIDS. Pediatric Guidelines For Infection Control of Human Immunodeficiency Virus (Acquired Immunodeficiency Virus) in Hospitals, Medical Offices, Schools, and Other Settings. *Pediatrics.* 1988;82:801–807
2. Centers for Disease Control. Education and foster care of children infected with HTLV III/LAV infection. *MMWR.* 1985;34:517–521
3. American Academy of Pediatrics, Committee on School Health and Committee on Infectious Diseases. School attendance of children and adolescents with human T lymphotropic virus III/lymphadenopathy-associated virus infection. *Pediatrics.* 1986;77:430–432
4. Ultmann MH, Belman AL, Ruff HA, et al. Developmental abnormalities in infants and children with acquired immune deficiency syndrome (AIDS) and AIDS Related Complex. *Dev Med Child Neurol.* 1985;27:563–571
5. Epstein LG, Sharer LR, Oleske JM, et al. Neurologic manifestations of human immunodeficiency virus infection in children. *Pediatrics.* 1986;78:678–687
6. Diamond GW, Cohen HJ. AIDS and developmental disabilities. *Prevention Update.* National Coalition in Preventing Mental Retardation, American Association of University Associated Programs, 8605 Cameron Street, Suite 406, Silver Spring, MD 20910
7. Belman AL, Diamond G, Lantos G, et al. Pediatric AIDS neurologic syndromes. *AJDC.* 1988;142:29–35
8. Diamond GW, Kaufman J, Belman AL, et al. Characterization of cognitive functioning in a subgroup of children with congenital HIV infection. *Arch Clin Neuropsychol.* 1987;2:245–256
9. American Academy of Pediatrics. Proceedings from A National Conference on Public Law 99-457: Physician Participation in the Implementation of the Law; November 19–21, 1988; Washington, DC
10. Sklaire MW, McInerny TK. Role of the pediatrician in school health. *Pediatr Rev.* 1990;12:69–70. Commentary
11. American Academy of Pediatrics, Committee on School Health. Acquired immunodeficiency syndrome education in schools. *Pediatrics.* 1988;82:278–280
12. American Academy of Pediatrics, Committee on Children with Disabilities and Committee on School Health. Children with health impairments in schools. *Pediatrics.* 1990;86:636–638
13. American Academy of Pediatrics. Concepts of school health programs. *AAP News.* 1985;1:16
14. American Academy of Pediatrics, Committee on School Health. Administration of medication in school. *Pediatrics.* 1984;74:433
15. American Academy of Pediatrics, Committee on School Health. Guidelines for urgent care in school. *Pediatrics.* 1990;86:999–1000
16. American Academy of Pediatrics. Home instruction. *AAP News.* 1985;1:16
17. Zlotnik JL. AIDS: helping families cope. Recommendations for meeting the psychosocial needs for persons with AIDS and their families. *Reports of the National Institutes of Mental Health,* November, 1987

AMERICAN ACADEMY OF PEDIATRICS

Guidelines for Human Immunodeficiency Virus (HIV)-Infected Children and Their Foster Families   (RE9237)

Task Force on Pediatric AIDS

STATEMENT OF THE PROBLEM

At the end of 1990, approximately 2786 cases of acquired immunodeficiency syndrome (AIDS) in children younger than 13 years of age had been reported to the Centers for Disease Control. Many more children are infected with the human immunodeficiency virus (HIV) but have milder or no apparent disease. The majority of young children have acquired their infection through perinatal transmission from HIV-infected mothers. A small minority have acquired their infection through blood transfusions received before 1985 when routine screening of the blood supply for HIV was initiated. Although many infants with perinatally acquired HIV infection will become symptomatic in the first year of life, a significant, but unknown, number of HIV-infected children are affected mildly or show minimal signs of infection for periods of up to 5 to 10 years.[1,2] There is evidence to suggest that antiretroviral treatment with Zidovudine prolongs survival, and it is hoped that early treatment will increase the interval between development of infection and symptoms and reduce the severity of symptoms.[3] Thus, children with HIV infection increasingly should be able to benefit from preschool and out-of-home child care programs. The social circumstances that may accompany HIV infection include (1) parents who have died or are too ill to care for their children; or (2) parents who are unable or unwilling to care for their children, most often as the result of continuing drug abuse. These situations frequently lead to the need for foster care or adoptive placement.

This statement makes recommendations regarding placement of HIV-infected children in adoptive or foster care homes and in child care settings.

BACKGROUND INFORMATION

Identification of HIV-infected children from birth to 15 to 18 months of age can be difficult because the presence of HIV-specific IgG antibody may be due to passive transfer from the HIV-infected mother.[4] By the time an infant is 15 to 18 months old, maternal antibody will have disappeared; therefore, the presence of antibody in a child this age indicates infection. Diagnosis is complicated further by the fact that a small number of infected infants fail to produce HIV-specific antibody, although most of them are symptomatic and some are quite ill. More definitive diagnostic techniques to accurately identify infection in an infant include tests for HIV antigenemia (p24 antigen), culture of the virus, detection of the viral genome by polymerase chain reaction, in vitro antibody production assays, and HIV-specific IgA antibody assays. However, the sensitivity and specificity of such testing still are being defined.[5-6] In children older than 15 to 18 months, the established antibody test (ie, Enzyme-Linked ImmunoSorbent Assay (ELISA)), followed by a confirmatory Western Blot Test is sufficient to detect most cases of HIV infection.

In adults and adolescents, HIV is transmitted most often through sexual intercourse (either homosexual or heterosexual) or through the sharing of needles and other injection equipment by intravenous drug users. Before the testing of blood for transfusions was initiated in 1985, a number of pediatric-age persons and adults were infected through transfusion of blood or blood products. Although anxieties about transmission of HIV in families or school settings exist, a number of studies have shown that HIV is not transmitted through casual or family-type contact, including hugging and kissing or sharing eating utensils, toilets, and bathing facilities with an infected person.[7] There has been no suggested transmission through sharing toys (even if they are placed in the mouth), by activities such as changing diapers, or through contamination of the child care environment with urine, stool, or vomitus. A few individuals, primarily health care workers, have become infected through injury with contaminated needles (risk is approximately 1 infection per 250 injuries), or under extremely rare circumstances, through direct contact of blood with the skin (most often broken skin). The risk of infection through direct contact with the skin can be diminished by following recommended precautions.

Biting is a common behavior in preschool child care settings. Although theoretically, biting is a possible mode of transmission of blood-borne illness, such as HIV infection or hepatitis B, actual transmission of HIV infection through biting has never been reported in a child care setting, and the risk of such transmission is thought to be negligible. Only one childhood case has been ascribed to a human bite; this possibility was not confirmed.[8,9]

PEDIATRICS (ISSN 0031 4005). Copyright © 1992 by the American Academy of Pediatrics.

Because HIV testing is not done routinely, there may be HIV-infected children in homes or child care settings who have not been identified because they are asymptomatic or have only mild symptoms. Because child care personnel will not always know whether a child has HIV infection or any other blood-borne disease (eg, hepatitis B), procedures that effectively protect against the transmission of blood-borne disease should be practiced universally in all child care settings. First, all wounds should be handled in a manner that minimizes direct contact between the blood and skin or mucous membranes of the care giver. In virtually all circumstances, the use of appropriate cloth barriers, such as thick toweling, to apply pressure or clean the wound is adequate. While some care givers may wish to use water-impervious gloves when tending to wounds, such is not required unless the care giver has a skin condition (eg, eczema, cuts, or abrasions) that results in nonintact skin.[10] Second, after all visible blood has been removed, all blood-contaminated environmental surfaces should be disinfected promptly with a fresh bleach solution diluted 1:100 (1 tablespoon bleach to 1 quart of water) or any chemical germicide that is approved by the Environmental Protection Agency for use as a hospital disinfectant. Regular washing of blood-contaminated clothing is sufficient.

Because children who have HIV infection or other chronic illnesses may be immunodeficient, it is important for their care givers to be informed of any infectious illnesses present in the child care setting that might compromise their health, such as measles or chickenpox. Because the child care providers may not know that there is an immunodeficient child present, child care programs should make it a policy to inform all families whenever a highly infectious illness such as measles or chickenpox has been identified in any child in the program.

Families are not required to inform child care providers that their child has HIV infection. However, it is advisable for child care providers to be informed about a child's HIV status to watch for signs of illness that may need medical attention and to address the child's and family's special emotional and social needs. In many jurisdictions this information can be divulged only with the written consent of the child's parent or legal guardian, and records of such information must be treated as confidential.

To promote foster care or adoptive placement, it is recommended that the HIV status of children born in high seroprevalence areas or in high-risk situations be determined when such testing would facilitate placement.[11] Courts should adopt methods for rapid processing of court orders to allow HIV testing of infants and children awaiting placement whenever such placement would be facilitated by testing. If the child is HIV-seronegative, which will be true in the majority of instances, the adopting or foster care home can be reassured that the child is not at risk for developing AIDS. If a child younger than 18 months of age is HIV-seropositive, the adoptive or foster care family should be informed fully about the risk that the child is truly infected (between 12.9% and 39%[12-14]), and the procedures by which that child should be followed up and/or treated. If infection has been documented, either by definitive testing (positive virus culture or p24 antigen test) or persistent antibody titers in a child older than the age of 18 months, the receiving family should be informed fully regarding the child's medical and psychosocial needs, and the community resources available for assisting HIV-infected children and their families. Also, foster care agencies should facilitate HIV testing of high-risk infants and children when medically indicated to promote appropriate medical treatment and follow up of those children who are HIV-seropositive.

RECOMMENDATIONS

Based on this information, the American Academy of Pediatrics makes the following recommendations.

1. There is no reason to restrict foster care or adoptive placement of children who have HIV infection to protect the health of other family members because the risk of transmission of HIV infection in family environments is negligible.

2. There is no need to restrict the placement of HIV-infected children in child care settings to protect child care personnel or other children in these settings, because the risk of transmission of HIV in child care environments is negligible.

3. Child care personnel need not be informed of the HIV status of a child to protect the health of care givers or other children in the child care environment. It should be noted that in some jurisdictions the child's diagnosis cannot be divulged without the written consent of the parent or legal guardian. Parents may choose to inform the child care provider of the child's diagnosis to support a request that the care giver observe the child closely for signs of illness that might require medical attention and assist the parents with the child's special emotional and social needs.

4. All child care settings should follow recommended universal precautions in the handling of blood or bloody fluids to minimize the possibility of transmission of any blood-borne disease.

5. All preschool child care programs routinely should inform all families whenever a highly infectious illness such as measles or chickenpox occurs in any child in that setting. This will help families protect their immunodeficient child.

6. To facilitate foster care or adoptive placement, courts should adopt methods for rapid processing of court orders to allow HIV testing of infants and young children whenever such testing would promote placement. Placement would be promoted most clearly when such court-ordered testing is pursued in areas of high seroprevalence or when the child comes from a high-risk setting.

Task Force on Pediatric AIDS, 1991 to 1992
Stanley A. Plotkin, MD, Chairman
Louis Z. Cooper, MD
Hugh E. Evans, MD
Norman C. Fost, MD, MPH
Sherrel L. Hammar, MD
Alfred Healy, MD
Renee Jenkins, MD
Gerald Merenstein, MD

Robert H. Pantell, MD
S. Kenneth Schonberg, MD
Gwendolyn B. Scott, MD
Martin W. Sklaire, MD

Liaison Representative
Martha F. Rogers, MD,
    Centers for Disease Control

Consultant
James R. Allen, MD, MPH,
    National AIDS Program Office

REFERENCES

1. Auger I, Thomas P, De-Gruttola V, et al. Incubation periods of paediatric AIDS patients. *Nature*. 1988;336:575–577
2. Burger H, Belman AL, Grimson R, et al. Long HIV-1 incubation periods and dynamics of transmission within a family. *Lancet*. 1990;336:134–136
3. McKinney RE Jr. Antiviral therapy for human immunodeficiency virus infection in children. *Pediatr Clin North Am*. 1991;38:133–151
4. American Academy of Pediatrics, Task Force on Pediatric AIDS. Perinatal human immunodeficiency virus infection. *Pediatrics*. 1988;82:941–944
5. Krivine A, Yakudima A, Le-May M, et al. A comparative study of virus isolation, PCR and antigen detection in children of mothers infected with human immunodeficiency virus. *J Pediatr*. 1990;116:372–376
6. Rogers MF, Ou CY, Kilbourne B, et al. Advances and problems in the diagnosis of human immunodeficiency virus infection in infants. *Pediatr Infect Dis J*. 1991;10:523–531
7. Rogers MF, White CR, Sanders R, et al. Lack of transmission of human immunodeficiency virus from infected children to their household contacts. *Pediatrics*. 1990;85:210–214
8. Wahn V, Kramer HH, Vott T, et al. Horizontal transmission of HIV infection between two siblings. *Lancet*. 1986;2:694
9. Shirley LR, Ross SA. Risk of transmission of human immunodeficiency virus by bite of an infected toddler. *J Pediatr*. 1989;114:425–427
10. American Academy of Pediatrics, Task Force on Pediatric AIDS. Pediatric guidelines for infection control of human immunodeficiency virus (acquired immunodeficiency syndrome virus) in hospital, medical offices, schools, and other settings. *Pediatrics*. 1988;82:801–807
11. American Academy of Pediatrics, Task Force on Pediatric AIDS. Infants and children with acquired immunodeficiency syndrome: placement in adoption and foster care. *Pediatrics*. 1989;83:609–612
12. Blanche S, Rouzioux C, Moscato MG, et al. A prospective study of infants born to women seropositive for HIV type 1. *N Engl J Med*. 1989;320:1643–1648
13. Ryder RW, Nsa W, Hassig SE, et al. Perinatal transmission of the HIV-type I to infants of seropositive women in Zaire. *N Engl J Med*. 1989;320:1637–1642
14. European Collaborative Study. Children born to women with HIV infection: natural history and risk of transmission. *Lancet* 1991;337:253–260

AMERICAN ACADEMY OF PEDIATRICS

Committee on Sports Medicine and Fitness

Human Immunodeficiency Virus [Acquired Immunodeficiency Syndrome (AIDS) Virus] in the Athletic Setting (RE9220)

Because athletes may bleed following trauma, they represent a theoretical risk to others if they are infected with the human immunodeficiency virus [HIV, acquired immunodeficiency syndrome (AIDS) virus]. Two questions have concerned coaches, athletic trainers, and school administrators: Should an athlete known to be infected with HIV be allowed to participate in competitive sports, and should the universal precautions recommended for health care workers[1] be used when handling athletes' blood and body fluids?

The risk of infection from skin exposure to the blood of a child or adolescent infected with HIV is unknown, but it is apparently minute and is much less than the risk of HIV infection by needlesticks from infected patients of approximately 1:250.[2] Although it is theoretically possible that transmission of HIV could occur in sports such as wrestling and football in which bleeding and skin abrasions are common, no such transmission has been reported in these sports. There is one report of possible transmission of HIV involving a collision between soccer players.[3] However, this report from Italy remains undocumented.

If an HIV-infected athlete would choose to pursue another sport, this possible risk to others would be avoided; but, in the absence of any proven risk, involuntary restriction of an infected athlete is not justified. Informing others of the athlete's status would probably lead to his or her exclusion due to inappropriate fear and prejudice and therefore should also be avoided. This advice must be reconsidered if transmission of HIV is found to occur in the sports setting. Athletes should also be made aware of the hazards of needle sharing for illicit drug use, including steroids.

Universal precautions adapted for the athletic setting are provided in Recommendation 6. Risk of exposure to a variety of infectious diseases is greater for coaches and trainers because of their interaction with many athletes. Competitors have extraordinarily low exposure rates. Coaches and athletic trainers should use these precautions if they are exposed repetitively to athletes' blood, because a rare athlete may have an HIV infection and because the athletic staff may not know this (as a result of the current practice of nondisclosure or because HIV-infected individuals may be asymptomatic and unaware of their infection).

The American Academy of Pediatrics recommends:

1. Athletes infected with HIV should be allowed to participate in all competitive sports. This advice must be reconsidered if transmission of HIV is found to occur in the sports setting.
2. A physician counseling a known HIV-infected athlete in a sport involving blood exposure, such as wrestling or football, should inform him of the theoretical risk of contagion to others and strongly encourage him to consider another sport.
3. The physician should respect a HIV-infected athlete's right to confidentiality. This includes not disclosing the patient's status of infection to the participants or the staff of athletic programs.
4. All athletes should be made aware that the athletic program is operating under the policies in Recommendations 1 and 3.

This statement has been approved by the Council on Child and Adolescent Health.

The recommendations in this publication do not indicate an exclusive course of treatment or serve as a standard of medical care. Variations, taking into account individual circumstances, may be appropriate.

5. Routine testing of athletes for HIV infection is not indicated.

6. The following precautions should be adopted:

a. Skin exposed to blood or other body fluids visibly contaminated with blood should be cleaned as promptly as is practical, preferably with soap and warm water. Skin antiseptics (eg, alcohol) or moist towelettes may be used if soap and water are not available.

b. Even though good hand-washing is an adequate precaution,[4] water-impervious gloves (latex, vinyl, etc) should be available for staff to use if desired when handling blood or other body fluids visibly contaminated with blood. Gloves should be worn by individuals with nonintact skin. Hands should be washed after glove removal.

c. If blood or other body fluids visibly contaminated with blood are present on a surface, the object should be cleaned with fresh household bleach solution made for immediate use as follows: 1 part bleach in 100 parts of water, or 1 tablespoon bleach to 1 quart water (hereafter called "fresh bleach solution"). For example, athletic equipment (eg, wrestling mats) visibly contaminated with blood should be wiped clean with fresh bleach solution and allowed to dry before reusing.

d. Emergency care should not be delayed because gloves or other protective equipment are not available.

e. If the care giver wishes to wear gloves and none are readily available, a bulky towel may be used to cover the wound until an off-the-field location is reached where gloves can be used during more definitive treatment.

f. Each coach and athletic trainer should receive training in first aid and emergency care and be provided with the necessary supplies to treat open wounds.

g. For those sports with direct body contact and other sports where bleeding may be expected to occur[5]:

1. If a skin lesion is observed, it should be cleansed immediately with a suitable antiseptic and covered securely[5].

2. If a bleeding wound occurs, the individual's participation should be interrupted until the bleeding has been stopped and the wound is both cleansed with antiseptic and covered securely or occluded.[5]

h. Saliva does not transmit HIV. However, because of potential fear on the part of those providing cardiopulmonary resuscitation, breathing (Ambu) bags and oral airways for use during cardiopulmonary resuscitation should be available in athletic settings for those who prefer not to give mouth-to-mouth resuscitation.

i. Coaches and athletic trainers should receive training in prevention of HIV transmission in the athletic setting; they should then help implement the recommendations suggested above.

COMMITTEE ON SPORTS MEDICINE
AND FITNESS, 1990 to 1991
Michael A. Nelson, MD, Chairman
Barry Goldberg, MD
Sally S. Harris, MD
Gregory L. Landry, MD
David M. Orenstein, MD
William L. Risser, MD

Liaison Representatives
Kathryn Keely, MD, Canadian
 Paediatric Society
Richard Malacrea, National Athletic
 Trainers Association
Judith C. Young, PhD, National
 Association for Sport and Physical Education

AAP Section Liaison
Arthur M. Pappas, MD, Section on
 Orthopaedics

REFERENCES

1. Centers for Disease Control. Update: recommendations for prevention of HIV transmission in health-care settings. *MMWR.* 1987;36(suppl 1):1–18
2. Henderson DK, Saah AJ, Zak BJ, et al. Risk of nosocomial infection with human T-cell lymphotropic virus type III/lymphadenopathy-associated virus in a large cohort of intensively exposed health care workers. *Ann Intern Med.* 1986;104:644–647
3. Torre D, Sampietro C, Ferraro G, Zeroli C, Speranza F. Transmission of HIV-1 infection via sports injury. *Lancet.* 1990;335:1105
4. Task Force on Pediatric AIDS, American Academy of Pediatrics. Pediatric guidelines for infection control of human immunodeficiency virus (acquired immunodeficiency virus) in hospitals, medical offices, schools, and other settings. *Pediatrics.* 1988;82:801–807
5. World Health Organization in collaboration with the International Federation of Sports Medicine. Consensus Statement from Consultation on AIDS and Sports. Geneva, Switzerland: January 16, 1989

AMERICAN ACADEMY OF PEDIATRICS

Task Force on Pediatric AIDS

Perinatal Human Immunodeficiency Virus Infection (RE 8128)

Infection with human immunodeficiency virus (HIV), the causative agent of acquired immunodeficiency syndrome (AIDS) has become a significant medical problem during the 1980s. Hundreds of infants and thousands of women have been reported to have AIDS. In addition, there are thousands more women infected with HIV, at risk for AIDS, and capable of transmitting HIV to their fetuses/infants if they become pregnant.

DEFINITIONS

Perinatal, the time period including pregnancy through 28 postnatal days; congenital (intrauterine) infection, infection acquired transplacentally; intrapartum infection, infection acquired during the time of delivery; postnatal infection, infection acquired after pregnancy and delivery; HIV infection, asymptomatic or symptomatic infection with HIV; AIDS, meeting the Centers for Disease Control definition for AIDS.

EPIDEMIOLOGIC FEATURES OF AIDS AND HIV

The primary risk factor for AIDS in infants is congenital (and possibly intrapartum) exposure to a mother infected with HIV. Other risks have included transfusion of blood or clotting factor concentrates. However, since the institution of routine testing of blood donors, these risks have become extremely small. Because the majority of women with AIDS (78%) are of childbearing age, it is important that the physician inquire about risk factors in women of childbearing age to provide optimal care and prevention of HIV transmission. The primary risk factors for AIDS in the reported cases in women are IV drug abuse (49%), hetero-

sexual transmission from a person known to be at risk of HIV infection (28%), and transfusion or clotting factor therapy before blood was screened in middle 1985 (11%).[1,2] Although the sex distribution of pediatric AIDS cases is relatively even (54% boys, 46% girls), the racial distribution of pediatric AIDS is uneven: blacks 54%, Hispanics 24%, whites 21%, and others 1%.[3]

RISKS AND MEANS OF CONGENITAL/INTRAPARTUM HIV INFECTION

The seroprevalence rate in an unselected population of childbearing women has been reported to range from 0.7/1,000 in New Mexico[4] to 20/1,000 in an inner New York City hospital.[5] In childbearing women who are IV drug abusers, the seropositive rate is 30%.[4] Hoff et al[6] reported seroprevalence rates in childbearing women in Massachusetts by type of hospital. They found 8/1,000 in the inner city hospitals, 2.6/1,000 in metropolitan hospitals, 2.2/1,000 in urban-suburban hospitals, 0.3/1,000 in suburban hospitals, and 1.2/1,000 in suburban-rural hospitals.[6] The rate for similar populations in New York City is 15.8/1,000 and for upstate New York it is 1.8/1,000.[4]

The risk of congenital or intrapartum transmission of HIV from an infected woman to her fetus or newborn depends on multiple factors that are not yet clearly defined. The best estimates of the risk for congenital or intrapartum transmission from an infected woman range from 30% to 50%, although reports of transmission have ranged from 0% to 65%.[7-11] The relevance of the timing of maternal infection, presence or absence of symptoms of AIDS in the mother, or other variables that influence transmission and infection in the fetus is unknown. Cesarean section has not been proven to be protective. Additional studies are necessary to define more precisely the risk and variables associated with perinatal transmission of HIV.

A few case reports suggest that women who were infected with HIV immediately postpartum (through blood transfusion) transmitted HIV to

---

PEDIATRICS (ISSN 0031 4005). Copyright © 1988 by the American Academy of Pediatrics.

their infants through breast-feeding.[12,13] Others have found that infants breast-fed as many as 7 months after birth did not become infected with HIV if they were born to women infected prepartum with HIV, suggesting that the relative risk of breast-feeding compared with intrauterine transmission is low.[8] Other types of postpartum transmission from a mother to her newborn (eg, physical affection such as touching and kissing) have not been documented.

DIAGNOSIS OF HIV INFECTION IN INFANTS

Because there is transplacental passage of maternal antibody to HIV in all infants born to seropositive mothers, the diagnosis of HIV infection in newborns is extremely difficult with currently available laboratory methods. Both the enzyme immunoassay (or enzyme-linked immunosorbent assay) and a confirmatory Western blot test are expected to be positive in the serum of both infected and uninfected infants born to a seropositive mother. Passive acquired HIV antibody decreases to undetectable levels in 50% of infants by 10 months, 75% of infants by 12 months, and most infants by 15 months. Unfortunately, some HIV-infected infants fail to elaborate HIV antibody and will, therefore, be HIV antibody negative but can be identified as HIV infected by viral culture and/or antigen detection. Thus, HIV seronegativity does not completely exclude congenital HIV infection.[8,14]

HIV infection is probable in an infant who, on serial specimens assayed by the same technique, has persistent or increasing titers of antibody to HIV or who demonstrates the appearance of new HIV-specific antibody bands on diagnostic tests such as Western blot or radioimmunoprecipitation assay. Additional tests currently under study include assays for HIV-specific IgM, HIV antigen, and viral nucleic acids and viral culture.[15,16] Positive viral culture of infant's blood or tissue is the definitive means of diagnosis but sensitivity is not established in infants. The sensitivity and specificity of the detection of HIV antigen and viral nucleic acids in infants is unknown.

CLINICAL FEATURES OF AIDS IN INFANTS

The incubation period of HIV infection in children may vary depending on the route of transmission. The majority of infants with perinatally acquired disease will appear normal at birth but within the first 24 months of life will have clinical illness. A small number of infected infants have remained asymptomatic for as many as 8 years.

Clinical features associated with HIV infection in infants include failure to thrive, generalized lymphadenopathy, hepatosplenomegaly, parotitis, persistent oral candidiasis, and chronic or recurrent diarrhea. Developmental disabilities and neurologic dysfunction are frequently seen. Bacterial infections with common organisms (*Streptococcus pneumonia* and *Haemophilus influenzae* type b) causing pneumonia, sepsis, meningitis, bone and joint infection, and otitis media are common and frequently recurrent. Lymphoid interstitial pneumonia has been reported in about 40% of infants and children with AIDS. Cardiomyopathy, hepatitis, and renal disease have also been described.

Craniofacial dysmorphic features have been reported in a small number of infants with HIV infection.[17-19] It is uncertain whether this is specifically due to HIV or whether other factors are involved.

Hyper-γ-globulinemia, particularly IgG, is usually present, although a few infected children may have hypo-γ-globulinemia.

Reported overall mortality in children with AIDS is 65% with the majority of deaths occurring during the first 24 months of life.

RISKS TO PERINATAL HEALTH CARE WORKERS (Appendix)

In health care workers, there are no known instances of HIV infection acquired through exposure to infants at delivery. The quantitative risk of acquisition of HIV infection by nonparenteral exposure has not been established, but it is clearly of a low magnitude. Nevertheless, medical history and examination do not reliably identify all mothers infected with HIV, and during delivery and initial care of the infant, health care workers are exposed to large amounts of maternal blood. In view of the utility of gloves in the prevention of other blood-borne diseases, and the low added costs involved, it is prudent for health care workers to use gloves for handling the placenta or the baby before he or she has been washed.[20,21]

RECOMMENDATIONS

1. Because the placenta and infant may be heavily contaminated with maternal blood, gloves should be used for handling the placenta or infant until the blood has been removed from the infant's skin. Hands should be washed immediately after gloves are removed and/or when skin surfaces are contaminated with blood.

2. Personnel assisting in the resuscitation of the newborn should use mechanical (adapted wall) suction equipment. Traps should be used in the line if mouth suction of the airway is performed in an emergency if mechanical suction is not available.

3. Infants of known seropositive mothers may be cared for in the normal nursery and do *not* require isolation in a private room or cubicle. Gloves should be worn for contact with blood or blood-containing fluids and for procedures that involve exposure to blood. Gloves are not required for prevention of HIV transmission while changing diapers in usual circumstances. Of course, hand washing after changing diapers is always required to reduce the transmission of other pathogens.[22]

4. Currently, a definitive determination that an infant <15 months of age is infected with HIV should be based on either (a) a diagnosis of AIDS based on Centers for Disease Control criteria or (b) a combination of antibody to HIV and a compatible immunologic profile and clinical course or (c) laboratory evidence of HIV in blood or tissues (culture or antigen detection).

5. In the United States and other countries where safe nutrition other than breast-feeding is available, HIV-infected mothers should be advised against breast-feeding their infants to avoid that possible route of HIV infection.

6. Presently, in most areas, prevalence of HIV infection in pregnant women does not warrant the cost of universal screening. However, serologic testing should be offered to pregnant women at increased risk for HIV infection. This may include routine screening of mothers (or newborns) in high seroprevalent areas. Counseling, guidance, and information should be offered to the woman who is seropositive or at high risk regarding the implications of a current or future pregnancy to both herself and the baby.

7. To prevent or better treat HIV infections there is a need to provide: (a) serologic surveys of anonymous specimens from infants to help define geographic prevalence of maternal HIV infection in areas where prevalence is unknown; (b) development and evaluation of new laboratory tests for the early identification of HIV infection in the newborn and young infant; (c) educational initiatives regarding AIDS, its transmission, and methods to prevent infection, including information concerning sexual and contraceptive behaviors; (d) counseling and easy access to drug treatment programs for individuals who are at increased risk for HIV infection secondary to such IV drug abuse; and (e) development and timely execution of carefully designed experimental protocols for the treatment of infants with HIV infection and its complications.

TASK FORCE ON PEDIATRIC AIDS,
1987–1988
Stanley A. Plotkin, MD, Chairman
Hugh E. Evans, MD

Norman C. Fost, MD, MPH
Gerald Merenstein, MD
S. Kenneth Schonberg, MD
Gwendolyn B. Scott, MD
Martin W. Sklaire, MD
Esther H. Wender, MD

Consultant
James R. Allen, MD, MPH

APPENDIX

The risk to health care workers of acquiring HIV infection in the perinatal setting will vary widely. The following analysis should help hospitals assess the risk, as well as the costs and benefits of implementing universal precautions on a routine basis.

Example 1: Low Prevalence Area

If the incidence of HIV infection in the maternal population is 1:1,000, then 1,000 deliveries would be required for a health care worker to be exposed to the HIV virus. Mere contact with such patients does not result in transmission; there must also be either a needlestick, blood coming in contact with mucous membranes, or abraded or cut skin. Not all needlesticks or blood on skin results in transmission: the risk of transmission to persons with needlesticks from infected patients is approximately 1:250.[23] Conclusive data for the risk of cutaneous exposure to perinatal fluids are not available. The risk of transmission for three estimates is as follows.

If transmission rate from blood fluids is:	No. of deliveries needed for transmission to occur	No. of years for transmission if 5,000 deliveries per year
1:100	100,000	20
1:250	250,000	50
1:1,000	1,000,000	200

Example 2: High Prevalence Area

If the incidence of HIV in the maternal population were 1:50, the following analysis would apply.

If transmission rate from blood fluids is:	No. of deliveries needed for transmission to occur	No. of years for transmission if 5,000 deliveries per year
1:100	5,000	1
1:250	12,500	2.5
1:1,000	50,000	10

The *benefits* of routine universal precautions, assuming they are 100% effective, will be prevention of one case of

HIV infection in a health care worker in the interval listed in the last column, as well as possible reduction of anxiety among the workers. There will be other benefits in preventing transmission of diseases that are more common than HIV infection, such as hepatitis B. The *costs* will include the direct costs of supplies and the added costs of disposal of such materials, which can be substantial.

REFERENCES

1. AIDS Weekly Surveillance Report—United States, AIDS Program, Centers for Disease Control, Feb 29, 1987
2. Guinan ME, Hardy A: Epidemiology of AIDS in women in the United States, 1981 through 1986. *JAMA* 1987;257:2039
3. Hopkins DR: AIDS in minority populations in the United States. *Public Health Rep* 1987;102:677
4. Centers for Disease Control: HIV infection in the United States. *MMWR* 1987;36:801
5. Landesman S, Minkoff H, Holman S, et al: Serosurvey of HIV infection in partuients: Implications for human immunodeficiency virus testing programs of pregnant women. *JAMA* 1987;258:2701
6. Berardi V, Hoff R, Wieblan B, et al: Seroprevalance of HIV among childbearing women: Estimation by testing samples of blood from newborns. *N Engl J Med* 1988;318:525
7. Semprini A, Vucetich A, Pardi G, et al: HIV infection and AIDS and newborn babies of mothers positive for HIV antibody. *Br Med J* 1987;294:610
8. Mok J, et al: Infants born to mothers seropositive for HIV. *Lancet* 1987;1:1164
9. Minkoff HL: Care of the pregnant woman infected with HIV. *JAMA* 1987;258:2714
10. Scott GB, Mastrucci M, Hutto S, et al: Pediatric HIV infection: Factors influencing case identification and prognosis, abstracted. *Pediatr Res* 1987;21:334A
11. Stewart G, Tyler J, Cunningham A, et al: Transmission of human T-cell lymphotropic virus type III (HTLV-III) by artificial insemination by donor. *Lancet* 1985;2:891
12. Ziegler JB, Cooper DA, Pekovish D, et al: Postnatal transmission of AIDS associated retrovirus from mother to infant. *Lancet* 1985;1:1980
13. Lepage P, et al: Postnatal transmission of HIV from mother to child. *Lancet* 1987;2:400
14. Borkowsky W, et al: HIV infections in infants negative for anti-HIV by ELISA. *Lancet* 1987;1:1168
15. Centers for Disease Control: Classification system for HIV infection in children under 13 years of age. *MMWR* 1987;36:225
16. Centers for Disease Control: Update: Serologic testing for antibody to HIV. *MMWR* 1988;36:833
17. Marion R, Hutcheon G, Wiznia A, et al: Fetal AIDS syndrome score. *Am J Dis Child* 1987;141:429
18. Bamji M, Iosub S, Stone RK, et al: More on human immunodeficiency virus embryopathy. *Pediatrics* 1987;80:512–516
19. Rogers MF, Thomas PA, Starcher ET, et al: Acquired immunodeficiency syndrome in children: Report of the Centers for Disease Control National Surveillance, 1982 to 1985. *Pediatrics* 1987;79:1008–1014
20. Centers for Disease Control: Recommendations for assisting in the prevention of perinatal transmission of human T-lymphocyte type III lymphadenopathy associated virus and acquired immunodeficiency syndrome. *MMWR* 1985;34:721
21. Centers for Disease Control: Recommendations for prevention of HIV transmission in healthcare settings. *MMWR* 1987;36(suppl 2):3S
22. American Academy of Pediatrics, AIDS Task Force: Pediatric guidelines infection control of HIV (AIDS Virus) in hospitals, medical offices, schools, and other settings. *Pediatrics* 1988;82:801–807
23. Henderson DK, Saah AJ, Szk BJ, et al: Risk of nosocomial infection with human T-cell lymphotrophic virus type III/lymphadenopathy associated virus in a large cohort of intensively exposed health care workers. *Ann Intern Med* 1986;104:644

AMERICAN ACADEMY OF PEDIATRICS

Perinatal Human Immunodeficiency Virus (HIV) Testing   (RE9239)

UNDER REVISION

Task Force on Pediatric AIDS

PERINATAL INFECTIONS

The primary route of human immunodeficiency virus (HIV) infection in infants is vertical transmission from HIV-infected mothers. This is of particular concern as the number of infected women and the number of children infected by perinatal transmission continue to increase rapidly. The number of perinatally acquired acquired immunodeficiency syndrome (AIDS) cases increased 17% in 1989 and 21% in 1990. Similarly, the number of heterosexually acquired AIDS cases increased 27% in 1989 and 40% in 1990. There is evidence that vertical transmission of HIV can occur in utero (congenital/transplacental, similar to rubella),[1,2] in the postpartum period (breast-feeding), and perhaps in the intrapartum period (similar to hepatitis B).[3] The relative frequency and efficiency of transmission during each of these periods remains uncertain. The best estimates of vertical transmission from an HIV-seropositive mother to the fetus range from 12.9% to 39%.[4-6] Although the risk of transmission appears to be increased in women who are symptomatic, this point is still unclear.[5] Preliminary information suggests that the presence of high levels of high-affinity/avidity antibodies to specific epitopes of the gp 120 of HIV may be protective and may decrease or prevent vertical transmission,[7-10] although others have not been able to confirm this finding.[11]

More detailed information on perinatal HIV infection,[12] and infection control[13] in pediatric HIV infection is available in previously published statements from the AAP Task Force on Pediatric AIDS.

SEROPREVALENCE

Anonymous seroprevalence data from newborn specimens are being collected in 44 states, Puerto Rico, and the District of Columbia. In some states, seroprevalence data are available by metropolitan area and/or by hospital of birth. Data from completed surveys are available from 38 states.[14] The overall US seroprevalence rate from these studies is 1.5/1000 although there is at least a tenfold geographic variation. Seroprevalence is highest in metropolitan areas, but it is increasing in small (50 000 to 100 000 population) urban and rural areas. It is important that anonymous seroprevalence testing be continued and expanded to monitor trends in maternal infection and estimates of future cases of pediatric HIV infections.

It should be noted that because the HIV antibody is transferred passively, testing of newborns provides only seroprevalence data for their mothers and does not prove infection of the newborn. New laboratory tests have been developed that may allow early (<6 months of age) identification of HIV infection in young infants. These tests include viral culture, polymerase chain reaction, in vitro antibody production, and detection of HIV-specific IgA or IgM antibodies (where the sensitivity has been enhanced by preabsorption with protein G).[15-22] At present, the use and interpretation of these tests should be limited to centers experienced in their evaluation.

ACCESS TO CARE

To justify a successful perinatal HIV counseling and testing program, women and their families must have access to care, including developmental screening and care programs for newborns. However, counseling and testing programs that may benefit the mother, fetus, and newborn cannot be delayed until access problems have been resolved completely. Services must be provided for the families as well as for individual HIV-infected women and should include psychosocial, behavioral, and clinical support. Care systems based on case management are particularly suited for the care of the family and must include counseling before and after testing. Assessment and reduction of risks should be part of initial counseling; however, testing should be offered to all and not based solely on self-identified risk factors.[23] Testing should be done only with pretest education, written informed consent, including the risks and benefits of testing for themselves and their infants, and posttest counseling on the meaning and implications of test results.

COSTS

The costs of perinatal HIV testing include direct costs such as counseling, obtaining informed consent, testing, follow-up and managing HIV-seropositive individuals, and indirect costs such as time and travel for those tested. There are other costs that are tangible although these are often difficult to quantify precisely. These costs include functional impairment due to psychologic distress while awaiting test results and after learning a test is positive, as well as adverse social consequences, including ostracism and loss of employment, with resulting loss of health insurance and other discrimination. Seropositive persons, including those who are false-positive, also experience adverse consequences associated with complications of medical treatment. However, because of the ex-

PEDIATRICS (ISSN 0031 4005). Copyright © 1992 by the American Academy of Pediatrics.

traordinary high specificity of the enzyme-linked immunosorbent assay and Western Blot tests (>99.9%) the positive predictive value will be high (and negative predictive value low), even in low-prevalence areas.

The costs of identifying persons who are HIV-seropositive are often compared with the savings associated with potentially reduced medical care expenses that may result with early intervention. In general, society is willing to pay for medical benefits, but not in excessive amounts, particularly when there are countless interventions of proven benefit for which resources could also be allocated. Therefore, it is customary to calculate the cost of achieving any specific outcome via cost-effectiveness analysis. Because both mother and infant benefit from perinatal HIV screening, costs for benefits to each need to be calculated according to documented efficacy (eg, cost for prolonged time the infant is free of infection, cost of hospitalization averted, cost per episode of pneumonia averted, cost per case identified, and cost of averting a subsequent infant at risk for HIV infection). Cost-effectiveness analysis is an essential part of the ongoing evaluation of the effectiveness and appropriateness of any testing program. Currently, the limited data about the efficacy of early treatment of HIV infection and the magnitude of psychological and social costs that accompany testing makes meaningful cost-effectiveness analysis an extraordinary problem that may become easier as our information base improves.

RISKS AND BENEFITS

A newborn who is HIV-seropositive has an HIV-seropositive mother; therefore, testing newborns using existing methods constitutes indirect maternal testing. As such, some women may be deterred from seeking prenatal care.

If identification of affected infants is associated with treatment, such testing is indicated. Therefore, short-term and long-term risks of treatment must be included in an assessment of risks of neonatal testing. This is of particular concern since at least two thirds of those infants who are HIV-seropositive will not be infected and may be exposed to risks of treatment that could possibly be harmful with no potential benefit.

Other risks of perinatal HIV testing are inherent in identifying any HIV-infected patient and are due primarily to anxiety and societal stigmatization.

The major medical benefits of perinatal testing and identification of HIV include a possible increase in life expectancy and better quality of life through the prevention, delay, or alleviation of HIV-related symptoms. Intravenous immunoglobulin has been shown to prolong the time of development of serious bacterial infection in HIV-infected children with CD4 (T4 helper) cell counts of greater than 200. Zidovudine has been shown to be beneficial in both adults[24-26] and children.[27,28] Pneumocystis carinii pneumonia prophylaxis using trimethoprim-sulfamethoxazole or aerosol pentamidine has been shown to be beneficial for HIV-infected adults, and trimethoprim-sulfa-

methoxazole is beneficial for children with leukemia.[29] While the benefit of such prophylaxis in HIV-infected infants and children has not been demonstrated in a controlled trial, Pneumocystis carinii pneumonia in infants often presents fulminantly and has a high mortality rate, particularly in infants younger than 12 months. Therefore, guidelines have been developed and prophylaxis is recommended for children based on age-adjusted CD4 cell counts.[30] To summarize, the potential medical benefits to mothers and infected newborns include: (1) reduced morbidity due to intensive health and developmental supervision, including chemoprophylaxis, Pneumocystis carinii pneumonia prophylaxis, prophylaxis and early treatment of bacterial infections, and appropriate immunizations; (2) an opportunity for early antiretroviral therapy[31-33]; (3) the provision of information regarding the risk of transmission from breast milk and the risk of vertical transmission in subsequent pregnancies; and (4) possible prevention of sexual transmission through education of the mother and father.

However, even when there are medical benefits for HIV-infected children, there may be other reasons to oppose mandatory testing. Mandatory (involuntary) testing may not necessarily be the most effective way to ensure that the largest number of children are tested.[34]

RECOMMENDATIONS

The American Academy of Pediatrics believes that counseling and testing for HIV should be available to both men and women (regardless of a woman's pregnancy status) and should be recommended to many of these individuals. HIV antibody testing programs should be voluntary and accompanied by appropriate education, counseling, informed consent, and confidentiality. In addition, testing programs and policies should reflect cultural, ethnic, and community values. A newborn who is HIV-seropositive has an HIV-seropositive mother; therefore, testing newborns using existing methods constitutes indirect maternal testing.

The following recommendations specifically address the perinatal period:

1. HIV testing should be routinely offered to all pregnant women and women of childbearing age throughout the United States by informing them of availability of counseling and testing.

2. HIV testing should be routinely recommended and encouraged for all pregnant women and women of childbearing age at increased risk of HIV infection because of high-risk behaviors or because they live in areas (state, metropolitan area, city, etc) with an HIV seroprevalence rate among pregnant women and newborns of 1:1000 or more.

3. Newborn testing should be routinely recommended and encouraged when mothers with known high-risk behaviors or from high-seroprevalence areas have not been tested.

4. HIV testing should be recommended and encouraged for abandoned infants and for infants otherwise in need of foster or adoptive care as needed to

facilitate placement and care. Courts should adopt methods for rapid processing of court orders to allow HIV testing of abandoned infants or those in foster care when follow-up adoption or initial placement may be facilitated by such testing.

5. Testing in the perinatal period should occur under specified policies which ensure retesting, education, informed consent, counseling, and follow-up criteria.

6. Anonymous seroprevalence surveys should be continued and expanded to identify hospital, city, and state seroprevalence information. These surveys are not a substitute for individual counseling and testing, but they provide important public health information.

7. Pilot studies of the benefits of perinatal testing, with careful evaluation of costs, are needed.

8. Specific tests for early diagnosis of HIV infection in infants must be developed further and made readily available to distinguish infection from passive transfer of maternal antibody.

9. Pediatricians or other primary pediatric care givers should be informed whenever an infant is born to a known HIV-seropositive mother so that appropriate care and follow-up testing can be done.

10. It is inappropriate to develop testing programs without addressing access to care. However, testing programs that may benefit the mother, fetus, and newborn cannot be delayed until access problems have been resolved completely.

11. The American Academy of Pediatrics opposes mandatory (involuntary) maternal and/or newborn testing at this time.

Task Force on Pediatric AIDS, 1991 to 1992
Stanley A. Plotkin, MD, Chairman
Louis Z. Cooper, MD
Hugh E. Evans, MD
Norman C. Fost, MD, MPH
Sherrel L. Hammar, MD
Alfred Healy, MD
Renee Jenkins, MD
Gerald Merenstein, MD
Robert H. Pantell, MD
S. Kenneth Schonberg, MD
Gwendolyn B. Scott, MD
Martin W. Sklaire, MD

Liaison Representative
Martha F. Rogers, MD, Centers for Disease Control

Consultant
James R. Allen, MD, MPH, National AIDS Program Office

REFERENCES

1. Hessami-Aghili AN, Spector SA. HIV Type 1 infection of human placenta. *J Virol.* 1991;65:2231–2236
2. Lewis SH, Reynolds-Kohler C, Fox HE, et al. HIV-1 in trophoblastic and villous Hofbauer cells and haematological precursors in eight-week fetuses. *Lancet.* 1990;335:565–568
3. Auger I, Thomas P, De Gruttola V, et al. Incubation periods for paediatric AIDS patients. *Nature.* 1988;336:575–577
4. Blanche S, Rouzioux C, Moscato MG, et al. A prospective study of infants born to women seropositive for HIV type 1. *N Engl J Med.* 1989; 320:1643

5. Ryder RW, Nsa W, Hassig SE, et al. Perinatal transmission of the HIV-type I to infants of seropositive women in Zaire. *N Engl J Med.* 1989; 320:1637–1642
6. European Collaborative Study. Children born to women with HIV infection: natural history and risk of transmission. *Lancet.* 1991; 337:253–260
7. Regaud M, Ming-Xia Z, Fidelia A, et al. Comparable anti-GP120 antibody titers in mothers delivering HIV infected and seroreverting infants. *Pediatr Res.* 1990;27:180A (1066)
8. Goedert JJ, Mendez H, Drummond JE, et al. Mother to infant transmission of HIV type I: association with prematurity or low anti-gp120. *Lancet.* 1989;1:1351–1354
9. Rossi P, Moschese V, Broliden PA, et al. Presence of maternal antibodies to HIV-I envelope glycoprotein gp120 epitopes correlates with the uninfected status of children born to seropositive mothers. *Proc Natl Acad Sci USA.* 1989;86:8055–8058
10. Devash Y, Calvelli TA, Wood DG, et al. Vertical transmission of human immunodeficiency virus is correlated with the absence of high-affinity/avidity maternal antibodies to the gp120 principal neutralizing domain. *Proc Natl Acad Sci USA.* 1990;87:3445–3449
11. Parekh BS, Schaffer N, Chou-Pong P, et al. Lack of correlation between maternal antibodies to V3 loop peptides of gp120 and perinatal HIV-1 transmission. *AIDS* 1991;5(10). In press
12. American Academy of Pediatrics, Task Force on Pediatric AIDS. Perinatal human immunodeficiency virus infection. *Pediatrics.* 1988;82: 941–943
13. American Academy of Pediatrics, Task Force on Pediatric AIDS. Pediatric guidelines for infection control of Human Immunodeficiency Virus (Acquired immunodeficiency virus) in hospitals, medical offices, schools, and other settings. *Pediatrics.* 1988;82:801–807
14. Gwinn M, Pappaioanou M, George JR, et al. Prevalence of HIV infection in childbearing women in the United States: surveillance using newborn blood samples. *JAMA.* 1991;265:1704
15. Krivine A, Yakudima A, Le May M, et al. A comparative study of virus isolation, PCR and antigen detection in children of mothers infected with HIV. *J Pediatr.* 1990;116:372–376
16. Johnson JP, Nair P, Hines SE, et al. Natural history and serologic diagnosis of infants born to HIV infected women. *AJDC.* 1989; 143:1147–1153
17. Schupbach J, Wunderli W, Kind C, et al. Frequent detection of HIV and IgG specific IgM and IgA antibodies in HIV+ cord blood sera: fine analysis by western blot. *AIDS* 1989;3:583–589
18. Broliden PA, Moschese V, Ljunggren K, et al. Diagnostic implications of specific IgG patterns of children born to HIV infected mothers. *AIDS.* 1989;3:577–582
19. Amadori A, De Rossi A, Chieco-Bianchi L, et al. Diagnosis of HIV-1 infection in infants: in vitro production of virus specific antibody in lymphocytes. *Pediatr Infect Dis J.* 1990;9:26–30
20. Rogers MF, Ou CY, Rayfield M, et al. Use of the PCR for early detection of the proviral sequences of HIV in infants born to seropositive mothers. *N Engl J Med.* 1989;320:1649
21. Martin NJ, Levy JA, Legg H, et al. Detection of infection with HIV Type 1 in infants by an anti-HIV immunoglobulin A assay using recombinant proteins. *J Pediatr.* 1991;178:354–358
22. Weiblen BJ, Lee FK, Cooper ER, et al. Early diagnosis of HIV infection by detection of IgA HIV antibodies. *Lancet.* 1990;335:988–990
23. Partridge JC, Sokal KB, Wong DF, et al. Maternal history does not predict perinatal HIV exposure. *Pediatr Res.* 1990;27:251A (1492)
24. Volberding PA, Lagakos SW, Koch MA, et al. Zidovudine in asymptomatic HIV infection: a controlled trial in persons with fewer than 500 CD4-positive cells per cubic millimeter. *N Engl J Med.* 1990; 322:941–949
25. Fischl MA, Richman D, Hansen N, et al. The safety and efficacy of zidovudine (AZT) in the treatment of subjects with mildly symptomatic human immunodeficiency virus type 1 (HIV) infection: a double-blind placebo-controlled trial. *Ann Intern Med.* 1990;112:727–737
26. Fischl MA, Richman D, Grieco M, et al. The efficacy of 3'-Azido-3'-deoxythymidine (azidothymidine) in the treatment of patients with AIDS and AIDS-related complex: a double-blind placebo-controlled trial. *N Engl J Med.* 1987;317:185–191
27. McKinney RE, Maha MA, Connor EN, et al. Multicenter trial of oral zidovudine in children with advanced human immunodeficiency virus disease. *N Engl J Med.* 1991;324:1018–1025
28. Pizzo PA, Eddy J, Fallon J, et al. Effect of continuous intravenous infusion of zidovudine (AZT) in children with symptomatic HIV infection. *N Engl J Med.* 1988;319:887–896
29. Centers for Disease Control. Guidelines for prophylaxis against Pneu-

mocystis carinii pneumonia for persons infected with HIV. *MMWR.* 1989;38(suppl):9

30. Centers for Disease Control. Guidelines for phophylaxis against Pneumocystis carinii pneumonia for children infected with human immunodeficiency virus. *MMWR.* 1991;40RR2:1

31. Ruprecht RM, O'Brien LG, Rossoni LD. Suppression of mouse viremia and retroviral disease by AZT. *Nature.* 1986;323:467–469

32. Tavares L, Roneker C, Johnston K, et al. AZT in feline leukemia virus infected cats, a model for therapy and prophylaxis of AIDS. *Cancer Res.* 1987;47:3190–3194

33. Sharpe AH, Jaenisch R, Ruprecht RM. Retroviruses and mouse embryos: a rapid model for neurovirulence and transplacental antiviral therapy. *Science.* 1987;236:1671–1674

34. Holtzman NA. *Proceed With Caution: Predicting Genetic Risks in the Recombinant DNA Era.* Baltimore, MD: John Hopkins University Press; 1989

Caring for Our Children: National Health and Safety Performance Standards: Guidelines for Out-of-Home Child Care Programs

Reprinted from
*Caring for Our Children: National Health and
Safety Performance Standards: Guidelines for
Out-of-Home Child Care Programs*
Copyright 1992
A Joint Collaborative Project of the
American Public Health Association
and the American Academy of Pediatrics

For information on ordering copies of
*Caring for Our Children: National Health and
Safety Performance Standards: Guidelines for
Out-of-Home Child Care Programs,*
contact:
American Academy of Pediatrics
Division of Publications
141 Northwest Point Blvd, PO Box 927
Elk Grove Village, IL 60009-0927
800/433-9016

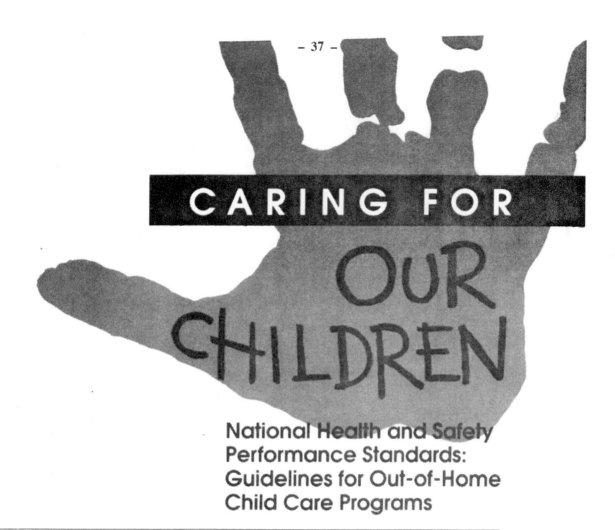

National Health and Safety Performance Standards: Guidelines for Out-of-Home Child Care Programs

6.7 Human Immunodeficiency Virus (HIV) Infection

Please note that if a staff member has no contact with the children, or with anything that the children come into contact with, these standards do not apply to that staff member.

ADMINISTRATIVE POLICIES ON HIV INFECTION

ID55. Human Immunodeficiency Virus (HIV)-infected children shall be admitted to child care providing their health, neurological development, behavior, and immune status are appropriate as determined on a case-by-case basis by qualified persons, including the child's health care provider, who are able to evaluate whether the child will receive optimal care in the specific facility being considered and whether an HIV-infected child poses a potential threat to others.

ID56. Information regarding a child whose immune system does not function properly to prevent infection, whatever the cause, shall be

No reported cases of HIV infection are known to have resulted from transmission in out-of-home child care. Although the risk of transmission of HIV infection to children in the child care setting appears to be extremely low, data do not exist that directly address this issue. Guidelines can most reasonably provide methods to reduce the risk of transmission of HIV infection to caregivers in out-of-home child care.

Since there are most likely HIV-infected children attending child care whose status is unknown, universal precautions should be adopted in

STANDARDS

available to those caregivers who need to know to protect the child against other infections. Accordingly, illnesses that occur among other children and staff in the facility shall be brought to the prompt attention of the parent of the child whose immune system does not function properly to prevent infection; such parent may elect to seek medical advice regarding continued participation of the child in the facility.

For additional information on administrative policies on HIV infection, see also *Confidentiality and Access to Records*, on p. 288.

PREVENTING TRANSMISSION OF HIV INFECTION

ID57. Child care personnel shall adopt universal precautions as outlined in *Prevention of Exposure to Blood*, on p. 74.

ID58. Caregivers shall be knowledgeable about routes of HIV transmission and about prevention of transmission.

ID59. HIV-infected adults with no symptoms of illness may care for children in facilities provided they do not have open skin sores or other conditions that would allow contact of their body fluids with children or other adults.

RATIONALE

caring for children in out-of-home child care.[78] The caregivers' need to know, however, does not require knowledge of the child's HIV status, since children whose immune systems do not function properly to prevent infections due to other acquired and congenital causes may also be in the facility.

See rationale in standard ID56, on p. 231.

Studies examining transmission of HIV support the concept that HIV is not a highly infectious agent.[79] The major routes of transmission are through sexual contact, through contact with blood, and from mother to child during the birth process. Several studies have shown that HIV-infected persons do not spread the HIV virus to other members of their households except through sexual contact. HIV has been isolated in very low volumes in saliva and urine. Transmission of hepatitis B virus (a virus very similar to HIV but more infectious) through saliva appears to be very uncommon. Isolated cases suggest that contact with blood from an HIV-infected individual is a possible mode of transmission. In these situations, the transmission appears most likely to have occurred through contact between nonintact skin and blood or blood-containing fluids.

On the basis of available data, there is no reason to believe that HIV-infected adults will transmit HIV in the course of their normal child care duties. Therefore, asymptomatic HIV-infected adults who do not have open, uncoverable skin sores or other conditions that would allow contact with

COMMENTS

Any child whose immune system does not function properly to prevent infection, however, will be suspected of having HIV and universal precautions will be implemented.

STANDARDS	RATIONALE	COMMENTS

their body fluids may care for children in facilities. However, immunosuppressed adults with acquired immunodeficiency syndrome (AIDS) may be more likely to acquire infectious agents from children and should consult with their own health care providers regarding the advisability of their continuing to work in a facility.[80]

PROTECTING HIV-INFECTED CHILDREN

ID60. Parents of an HIV-infected child shall be notified immediately if the child has been exposed to chicken pox, Tb, or measles through other children in the facility.

Children who are infected with HIV often have immune systems that do not function properly to prevent infections. Children with immunosuppression for multiple other reasons are at increased risk for severe complications from infections with chicken pox, CMV, Tb, and measles virus.[81] Available data indicate that measles infection is a more serious illness in HIV-infected children than in noninfected children. The first deaths due to measles in the United States reported to the CDC after 1985 were in HIV-infected children.[82]

ID61. A child whose immune system does not function properly to prevent infection and who is exposed to measles or chicken pox shall be referred immediately to his/her health care provider to receive the appropriate preventive measure (immune globulin) following exposure.

See rationale for standard ID60.

ID62. The decision to readmit the exposed child to the facility shall be made jointly by the center director or large or small family home caregiver, the family, and the child's health care provider.

See rationale for standard ID60.

ID63. Caregivers known to be HIV-infected shall be notified immediately if they have been exposed to chicken pox, Tb, or measles through children in the facility; they shall receive an appropriate preventive measure (immune globulin) after exposure if exposed to measles or chicken pox; and their return to work after exposure shall be determined jointly by the center director or large or small family home caregiver and the health care provider for the HIV-infected caregiver.

See rationale for standard ID60.

References

1. Recommendations of the Immunization Practices Advisory Committee (ACIP). Update: prevention of *Haemophilus influenzae* type b disease. *MMWR*. 1988;37:13–16.

2. American Academy of Pediatrics Committee on Infectious Disease: *Haemophilus influenzae* type b conjugate vaccine. *Pediatrics*. 1988;81:908–911.

3. Schlech WF, Ward JI, Band JD, et al. Bacterial meningitis in the United States, 1978 through 1981. *JAMA*. 1985;253:1749–1754.

4. Cochi SL, Fleming DW, Hightower AW, et al. Primary invasive *Haemophilus influenzae* type b disease: a population-based assessment of risk factors. *J Pediatr*. 1986;108:887–896.

5. Osterholm MT, Pierson LM, White KE, et al. The risk of a subsequent transmission of *Haemophilus influenzae* type b disease among children in day care. *N Engl J Med*. 1987;316:1–5.

6. Murphy TV, Clements JF, Breedlove JA, et al. Risk of subsequent disease among day-care contacts of patients with systemic *Haemophilus influenzae* type b disease. *N Engl J Med*. 1987;316:5–10.

7. Band JD, Fraser DW, Ajello G, et al. Prevention of *Haemophilus influenzae* type b disease. *JAMA*. 1984;253:2381–2386.

8. Makintubee S, Istre GR, Ward JI. Transmission of invasive *Haemophilus influenzae* type b disease in day care settings. *J Pediatr*. 1987;111:180–186.

9. Fleming DW, Leibenhaut MH, Albanes D, et al. Secondary *Haemophilus influenzae* type b in day-care facilities: risk factors and prevention. *JAMA*. 1985;254:509–514.

10. Murphy TV, McCracken GH, Moore BS, et al. *Haemophilus influenzae* type b disease after rifampin prophylaxis in a day care center: possible reasons for its failure. *Pediatr Infect Dis*. 1983; 2:193–198.

11. Fraser DW, Geil CC, Feldman RA. Bacterial meningitis in Bernalillo County, New Mexico. A comparison with three other American populations. *Amer J Epidemiol*. 1974;100:29–34.

12. Jacobson JA, Felice GA, Holloway JT. Meningococcal disease in day-care centers. *Pediatrics*. 1977;59:299–300.

13. Centers for Disease Control. Pertussis surveillance—United States, 1984 and 1985. *MMWR*. 1987;36:168–171.

14. Bass JE. Pertussis: current status of prevention and treatment. *Pediatr Infect Dis*. 1985;4:614–619.

15. Smith TD, Wilkinson V, Kaplan EL. Group A streptococcus-associated upper respiratory tract infections in a day-care center. *Pediatrics*. 1989;83:380–384.

16. Kaplan EL. Personal communication, March 21, 1989.

17. Kaplan EL, Hill HR. Return of rheumatic fever: consequences, implications, and needs. *J Pediatr*. 1987;111:244–246.

18. Denny FW, Collier AM, Henderson FW. Acute respiratory infections in day care. In: Osterholm MT, Klein JO, Aronson SS, Pickering LK, eds. *Infectious Diseases in Child Care: Management and Prevention*. Chicago, Ill: University of Chicago Press; 1987; 15–20.

19. Dingle JH, Badger GF, Jordan WS. *Illness in the Home: A Study of 25,000 Illnesses in a Group of Cleveland Families*. Cleveland, Ohio: Press of Case Western Reserve University; 1964.

20. Fleming DW, Cochi SL, Hightower AW, Broome CV. Childhood upper respiratory tract infections: to what degree is incidence affected by day-care attendance? *Pediatrics*. 1987;79:55–60.

21. Wald ER, Dashefsky B, Byers C, et al. Frequency and severity of infections in day care. *J Pediatr*. 1988; 112:540–546.

22. Anderson LJ, Parker RA, Stricas RS, et al. Day-care attendance and hospitalization for lower respiratory tract illness. *Pediatrics*. 1988;82:300–308.

23. Gala CL, Hall CB, Schnable KC, et al. The use of eye-nose goggles to control nosocomial respiratory syncytial virus infection. *JAMA*. 1986;256:2706.

24. St. Gene J, Pickering L, Granoff D. Symposium—Day care diseases: does day care make respiratory illness worse? *Contemp Pediatr*. 1986;3:22–42.

25. Trumpp C. Management of communicable diseases in day care centers. *Pediatr Annals*. 1983;12(3).

26. Black RE, Dykes AC, Anderson KD, et al. Handwashing to prevent diarrhea in day care centers. *Am J Epidemiol*. 1981;113:445–451.

27. Aronson SS, Aiken LS. Compliance of child care programs with health and safety standards: impact of program evaluation and advocate training. *Pediatrics*. 1980;65:318–325.

28. Bartlett AV, Jarvis BA, Ross V, et al. Diarrheal illness among infants and toddlers in day care centers: effects of active surveillance and staff training without subsequent monitoring. *Amer J Epidemiol*. 1988;127:808–817.

29. Sullivan P, Woodward WE, Pickering LK, et al. A longitudinal study of the occurrence of diarrheal disease in day care centers. *Amer J Public Health*. 1984;74:987–991.

30. Pickering LK, Evans DG, DuPont HL, et al. Diarrhea caused by *Shigella*, rotavirus, and *Giardia* in day care centers: prospective study. *J Pediatr*. 1981;99:51–56.

31. Bartlett AV, Moore M, Gary GW, et al. Diarrheal illness among infants and toddlers in child day care centers. *J. Pediatr*. 1985;107:495–502.

32. Pickering LK, Hadler SC. Management and prevention of infectious diseases in day care. In: Feigin RD, Cherry JD, eds. *Textbook of Pediatric Infectious Diseases*. Philadelphia, Pa: WB Saunders Co; 1987. 2343–2361.

33. Hadler SC, Erben JJ, Francis DP, et al. Risk factors for hepatitis A in day care centers. *J Infect Dis*. 1982; 145:255–261.

34. Hadler SC, Webster HM, Erben JJ, et al. Hepatitis A in day care centers: a community-wide assessment. *N Engl J Med.* 1980;302:1222–1227.

35. Pickering LK, Woodward WE, DuPont HL, et al. Occurrence of *Giardia lamblia* in children in day care centers. *J Pediatr.* 1984;104:522–526.

36. Pickering LK, Bartlett AV, Reves RR, Morrow A. Asymptomatic rotavirus before and after rotavirus diarrhea in children in day care centers. *J Pediatr.* 1988; 112:361–365.

37. Keswick BH, Pickering LK, DuPont HL, et al. Survival and detection of rotavirus on environmental surfaces in day care centers. *Appl Environ Microbiol.* 1983;46:813–816.

38. Kim K, DuPont HL, Pickering LK. Outbreaks of diarrhea associated with *Clostridium difficile* and its toxin in day care centers: evidence of person-to-person spread. *J Pediatr.* 1983;102:376–382.

39. Petersen JJ, Bressler GK. Design and modification of the day care environment. *Rev Infect Dis.* 1986; 8:618–621.

40. Weniger BG, Ruttenber J, Goodman RA. Fecal coliforms on environmental surfaces in two day care centers. *Appl Environ Microbiol.* 1983;45: 733–735.

41. Pickering, LK, Bartlett AV, Woodward WE. Acute infectious diarrhea among children in day care: epidemiology and control. *Rev Infect Dis.* 1986; 8:539–547.

42. Hinman AR. Vaccine-preventable diseases and child day care. *Rev Infect Dis.* 1986; 8:573–583.

43. Markowitz LE, Preblud SR, Orenstein, WA. Patterns of transmission in measles outbreaks in the United States, 1985–1986. *N Engl J Med.* 1989;320:75–81.

44. Centers for Disease Control. Measles—United States, 1986. *MMWR.* 1987;36:301–305.

45. Centers for Disease Control. Mumps—United States, 1985–1988. *MMWR.* 1989; 38:101–105.

46. Recommendations of the Immunization Practices Advisory Committee (ACIP). General recommendations on immunization. *MMWR.* 1989;38:205–227.

47. American Academy of Pediatrics. *Report of the Committee on Infectious Diseases.* 21st edition. Elk Grove Village, Ill: American Academy of Pediatrics; 1988.

48. Centers for Disease Control. Rubella and congenital rubella syndrome—United States, 1985–1988. *MMWR.* 1989;38:173–178.

49. Recommendations of the Immunization Practices Advisory Committee (ACIP). Adult immunizations. *MMWR.* 1984;33S:1S–68S.

50. Kohl S. Postnatal herpes simplex virus infections. In: Feigin RD, Cherry JD, eds. *Textbook of Pediatric Infectious Diseases.* Philadephia, Pa: WB Saunders Co; 1987:1577–1601.

51. Juretic M. Natural history of herpetic infection. *Helv Paedatr Acta.* 1966;21:356–368.

52. Paryani SG, Arvin AM. Intrauterine infection with varicella-zoster virus after maternal varicella. *N Engl J Med.* 1986;314:1542–1546.

53. Prevalence of cytomegalovirus excretion from children in five day care centers—Alabama. *MMWR.* 1985;34:49–51.

54. Stagno S, Pass RF, Dworsky ME, Alford CA. Maternal cytomegalovirus infection and perinatal transmission. In: Knox GE, ed. *Clinical Obstetrics and Gynecology.* 1982:25:563–576.

55. Stagno S, Pass RF, Dworsky MD, et al. Congenital cytomegalovirus infection: the relative importance of primary and recurrent maternal infection. *N Engl J Med.* 1982;306:945–949.

56. Pass RF, August AM, Dworsky M, et al. Cytomegalovirus infection in a day care center. *N Engl J Med.* 1982;307:477–479.

57. Hutto C, Ricks RE, Pass RF. Prevalence of cytomegalovirus excretion from children in five day care centers. *JAMA.* 1985;253:1236–1240.

58. Hutto C, Ricks R, Garvie M, Pass RF. Epidemiology of cytomegalovirus infections in young children: day care vs. home care. *Pediatr Infect Dis.* 1985; 4:149–152.

59. Adler SP. The molecular epidemiology of cytomegalovirus transmission among children attending a day care center. *J Infect Dis.* 1985;152:760–769.

60. Pass RF, Hutto SC, Reynolds DW, et al. Increased frequency of cytomegalovirus infection in children in group day care. *Pediatrics.* 1984;74:121–126.

61. Pass RF, Hutto C. Group day care and cytomegaloviral infections of mothers and children. *Rev Infect Dis.* 1986;8:599–605.

62. Adler SP. Molecular epidemiology of cytomegalovirus: evidence for viral transmission to parents from children infected at a day care center. *Pediatr Infect Dis.* 1986;5:315–318.

63. Grillner L, Strangert K. Restriction endonuclease analysis of cytomegalovirus DNA from strains isolated in day care centers. *Pediatr Infect Dis.* 1986;5:184–187.

64. Hutto C, Little A, Ricks R, et al. Isolation of cytomegalovirus from toys and hands in a day care center. *J Infect Dis.* 1986;154:527–530.

65. Murph JR, Bale JF, Murray JC, et al. Cytomegalovirus transmission in a midwest day care center: possible relationship to child care practices. *J Pediatr.* 1986;109:35–39.

66. Yeager AS. Transmission of cytomegalovirus to mothers by infected infants: another reason to prevent transfusion-acquired infections. *Pediatr Infect Dis.* 1983;2:295–297.

67. Spector SA, Spector DH. Molecular epidemiology of cytomegalovirus infection in premature twin infants and their mother. *Pediatr Infect Dis.* 1982;1:403–409.

68. Pass RF, Hutto C, Ricks R, Cloud GA. Increased rate of cytomegalovirus infection among parents of children attending day care centers. *N Engl J Med.* 1986;314:1414–1418.

69. Pass RF, Hutto C, Cloud G. Day care workers and cytomegalovirus infection. *Clin Res.* 1988;36:65A.

70. Adler SP. Risk of cytomegalovirus infection among women employed at day care centers. *Pediatr Res.* 1988;23:362A.

71. Stagno RF, Little EA, Stagno S, et al. Young children as a probable source of maternal and congenital cytomegalovirus infection. *N Engl J Med.* 1987;316:1366–1370.

72. Stagno S, Pass RF, Cloud C, et al. Primary cytomegalovirus infection in pregnancy: incidence, transmission to the fetus and clinical outcome in two populations of different economic backgrounds. *JAMA.* 1986;256:1904–1908.

73. Ahlfors K, Ivarson SA, Harris S, et al. Congenital cytomegalovirus infection and disease in Sweden and the relative importance of primary and secondary maternal infections. Primary findings from a prospective study. *Scand J Inf Dis.* 1984;16:129–137.

74. Griffiths PD, Baboonian C. A prospective study of primary cytomegalovirus infection during pregnancy: final report. *Br J Obstet Gynecol.* 1984;91:307–315.

75. Stagno S, Reynolds DW, Huang E-S, et al. Congenital cytomegalovirus infection. *N Engl J Med.* 1977;296:1254–1258.

76. Shapiro CN, McCaig LF, Genesheimer KF, et al. Hepatitis B virus transmission between children in day care. *Pediatr Infect Dis.* 1989;8:870–875.

77. Shapiro ED. Lack of transmission of hepatitis B in a day care center. *J Pediatr.* 1987;110:90–92.

78. Task Force on Pediatric AIDS. Pediatric guidelines for infection control of human immunodeficiency virus (acquired immunodeficiency virus) in hospitals, medical offices, schools and other settings. *Pediatrics.* 1988;82:801–808.

79. MacDonald KL, Danila RN, Osterholm MT. Infection with human T-lymphotrophic virus type III/lymphadenopathy-associated virus: considerations for transmission in the child day care setting. *Rev Infect Dis.* 1986;8:606–612.

80. Centers for Disease Control. Education and foster care of children infected with human T-lymphotrophic virus type III/lymphadenopathy-associated virus. *MMWR.* 1985;34:517–521.

81. Immunization of children infected with human immunodeficiency virus—supplementary ACIP statement. *MMWR.* 1988;37:181–183.

82. Measles in HIV-infected children, United States. *MMWR.* 1988;37:183–186.

OSHA: Materials to Assist the Pediatric Office in Implementing the Bloodborne Pathogen, Hazard Communication, and Other OSHA Standards

Reprinted from *OSHA: Materials to Assist the Pediatric Office in Implementing the Bloodborne Pathogen, Hazard Communication, and Other OSHA Standards,* 2nd edition
Copyright 1994 by the American Academy of Pediatrics

For information on ordering copies of
OSHA: Materials to Assist the Pediatric Office in Implementing the Bloodborne Pathogen, Hazard Communication, and Other OSHA Standards, contact:
American Academy of Pediatrics
Division of Publications
141 Northwest Point Blvd, PO Box 927
Elk Grove Village, IL 60009-0927
708/228-5005

Introduction

The Occupational Safety and Health Administration (OSHA) standard 1910.1030, Occupational Exposure to Bloodborne Pathogens, is designed to protect health care workers from contamination due to potentially infectious materials that may be present in the workplace. Since any exposure to blood poses a serious health risk in a health care setting, the standard covers employees who may be reasonably anticipated to come into contact with human blood and other potentially infectious material in order to perform their jobs. The standard mandates that each health care facility institute engineering controls, work practices, and personal protective equipment that, coupled with employee training, will reduce on-the-job risks for all employees exposed to blood. Meeting these requirements is not optional. It is essential to prevent illness and chronic infection among health care workers and to comply with the law.

The OSHA Hazard Communication Standard, 1910.1200, has been expanded to include non-manufacturing industries, including physicians offices. The standard mandates that employers design a Hazard Communication Program and communicate it to employees through training sessions. This standard is required of all employers in an effort to ensure the safety of employees through identification of and protection from hazardous chemicals.

The first part of this AAP kit deals with the standard regulating occupational exposure to bloodborne pathogens, and consists of the following: a model exposure control plan, worksheets to guide you through the exposure control plan and to assist you in completing it, information and training guidelines, a key summary of the standard's provisions, fact sheets, and a listing of other resources to consult for information on the standard. The second part of this AAP kit deals with the standard regulating hazard communication and consists of the following: steps for compliance, a sample Hazard Communication Program, samples of required forms, and a copy of the amended standard. The third part of this AAP kit contains information on OSHA's posting, recordkeeping, and reporting requirements, information on other OSHA standards and state/local medical waste regulations, and a list of OSHA offices.

The standards require employers who have employees who are, or who may be, exposed to bloodborne pathogens and hazardous chemicals to develop a written exposure control plan and a written Hazard Communication Program. The AAP model exposure control and accompanying worksheets, as well as the sample Hazard Communication Program and sample forms, are designed to guide you through the standards and facilitate bringing your facility into compliance with the standards. It may be necessary to modify the AAP model plan and sample policy to address the needs of your particular practice. You may also wish to have your specific plan reviewed by your attorney to ensure that you are fully complying with the standards. The training and information guidelines identify information about the standards that must be conveyed to all employees at risk of occupational exposure to bloodborne pathogens and hazardous chemicals.

The Academy has designed this kit to both assist you in complying with standards and to alleviate your concerns regarding their implementation in your office. However, none of the information provided in this kit is intended to absolve you of your responsibility to comply with the OSHA standards.

Introduction to Bloodborne Pathogen Standard

In December 1991, the Occupational Safety and Health Administration ("OSHA") issued regulations that are designed to reduce employees' occupational exposure to bloodborne pathogens. According to the OSHA standard, all employers with employees who may be exposed to bloodborne pathogens or other potentially infectious materials must develop a written exposure control plan.

The exposure control plan must (1) identify employees who have or who the employer anticipates will have occupational exposure to bloodborne pathogens, (2) provide precautions and facility practice controls to reduce occupational exposure, (3) provide cleaning procedures for the facility and certain employee clothing, (4) provide protective equipment to employees, (5) provide vaccinations to employees and medical evaluations of employees who have had an exposure incident (eg, a needlestick), and (6) provide disposal procedures for certain types of waste.

Occupational exposure means reasonably anticipated skin, eye, mucous membrane, or parenteral contact with blood or other potentially infectious materials that may result from the performance of the employee's duties. Other potentially infectious material includes the following: (1) human body fluids: semen, vaginal secretions, cerebrospinal fluid, synovial fluid, pleural fluid, pericardial fluid, peritoneal fluid, amniotic fluid, saliva in dental procedures, any body fluids visibly contaminated with blood, and all body fluids in situations where it is difficult or impossible to differentiate between body fluids; (2) any unfixed tissue or organ (other than intact skin) from a human (living or dead); and, (3) human immunodeficiency virus (HIV) - containing cell or tissue cultures, organ cultures, and HIV or hepatitis B virus (HBV) - containing culture medium or other solutions as well as blood, organs, or other tissues from experimental animals infected with HIV or HBV.

The plan must be easily accessible to employees and to the Assistant Secretary of Labor of Occupational Safety and Health, the Director of the National Institute for Occupational Safety and Health and the Director of the US Department of Health and Human Services. If the plan is maintained solely on a computer, employees must be trained to operate the computer. A copy of the plan must be provided within 15 working days of the request.

The plan must be updated annually to reflect modifications in tasks or procedures that may result in occupational exposure and whenever a new procedure or task that affects occupational exposure is added or modified.

The Academy has developed this model exposure control plan to assist you in complying with the OSHA regulations. The AAP model plan is intended to be a guide that you can use to develop your own exposure control plan. It is not intended to absolve you of the responsibility to know and comply with the OSHA regulations. In addition, the recommendations in this publication do not indicate an exclusive course of treatment or serve as a standard of medical care. If you need additional space to complete any portion of the plan, please copy the appropriate pages and append them to the plan.

Fact Sheet

OSHA Bloodborne Pathogens Final Standard
Summary of Key Provisions

Purpose: Limits occupational exposure to blood and other potentially infectious materials since any exposure could result in transmission of bloodborne pathogens that could lead to disease or death.

Scope: Covers *all employees who* could be "reasonably anticipated" as the result of performing their job duties *face contact with blood* and other potentially infectious materials. OSHA has not attempted to list all occupations in which exposures could occur. "Good Samaritan" acts such as assisting a co-worker with a nosebleed would not be considered occupational exposure.

Infectious materials include semen, vaginal secretions, cerebrospinal fluid, synovial fluid, pleural fluid, pericardial fluid, peritoneal fluid, amniotic fluid, saliva in dental procedures, any body fluid visibly contaminated with blood and all body fluids in situations in which it is difficult or impossible to differentiate between body fluids. They also include any unfixed tissue or organ other than intact skin from a human (living or dead) and human immunodeficiency virus (HIV) - containing cell or tissue cultures, organ cultures, and HIV- or hepatitis B (HBV) - containing culture medium or other solutions as well as blood, organs, or other tissues from experimental animals infected with HIV or HBV.

Exposure Control Plan: Requires employers to *identify, in writing,* tasks and procedures as well as job classifications *where occupational exposure to blood and other potentially infectious materials occurs* -- without regard to personal protective clothing and equipment. It must also set forth the *schedule for implementing other provisions* of the standard and specify the procedure for evaluating circumstances surrounding exposure incidents. The plan must be accessible to employees and available to OSHA. Employers must review and update it at least annually -- more often if necessary to accommodate workplace changes.

Methods of Compliance: Mandates *universal precautions* (treating body fluids/materials as if infectious) *emphasizing engineering and work practice controls.* The standard stresses handwashing and requires employers to provide facilities and ensure that employees use them following exposure to blood. It sets forth procedures to minimize needlesticks, minimize splashing and spraying of blood, ensure appropriate packaging of specimens and regulated wastes, and decontaminate equipment or label it as contaminated before shipping to servicing facilities.

Employers must provide, at no cost, and require employees to use, appropriate *personal protective equipment* such as gloves, gowns, masks, mouthpieces, and resuscitation bags and must clean, repair and replace these when necessary. Gloves are not necessarily required for routine phlebotomies in volunteer blood donation centers but must be made available to employees who want them.

The standard requires a *written schedule for cleaning* and decontaminating exposure areas, and identification of the methods for cleaning and decontamination to be used. The standard specifies methods for disposing of contaminated sharps and sets forth standards for containers for these items and other regulated waste. Further, the standard includes provisions for handling contaminated laundry to minimize exposures.

HIV and HBV Research Laboratories and Production Facilities: Calls for these facilities to follow *standard microbiological practices* and specifies additional practices intended to minimize exposures of employees working with concentrated viruses and reduce the risk of accidental exposure for other employees at the facility. These facilities must include required containment equipment and an autoclave for decontamination of regulated waste and must be constructed to limit risks and enable easy clean up. *Additional training and experience requirements* apply to workers in these facilities.

Hepatitis B Vaccination: Requires vaccinations to be made *available to all employees who have occupational exposure to blood* or other potentially infectious materials within 10 working days of assignment, at no cost, at a reasonable time and place, under the supervision of licensed physician/ licensed healthcare professional and according to the latest recommendations of the U.S. Public Health Service (USPHS). *Pre- screening may not be required* as a condition of receiving the vaccine. Employees must sign a *declination form* if they choose not to be vaccinated, but may later opt to receive the vaccine at no cost to the employee. Should booster doses later be recommended by the USPHS, employees must be offered them.

Postexposure Evaluation and Follow-up: Specifies procedures to be made *available to all employees who have had an exposure incident* plus any laboratory tests must be conducted by an accredited laboratory at no cost to the employee. Follow-up must include a *confidential medical evaluation* documenting the circumstances of exposure, identifying and testing the source individual if feasible, testing the exposed employee's blood if he/she consents, postexposure prophylaxis, counseling and evaluation of reported illnesses. Health care professionals must be provided specified information to facilitate the evaluation and their written opinion on the need for hepatitis B vaccination following the exposure. Information such as the employee's ability to receive the hepatitis B vaccine must be supplied to the employer. All diagnoses must remain confidential.

Hazard Communication: Requires *warning labels* including the *orange or orange-red biohazard symbol* affixed to containers of regulated waste, refrigerators and freezers, and other containers that are used to store or transport blood or other potentially infectious materials. *Red bags* or containers *may be used* instead of labeling. When a facility uses universal precautions in its handling of all specimens, labeling is not required within the facility. Likewise, when all laundry is handled with universal precautions, the laundry need not be labeled. Blood that has been tested and found free of HIV or HBV and released for clinical use, and regulated waste that has been decontaminated need not be labeled.

Signs must be used to *identify restricted areas* in HIV and HBV research laboratories and production facilities.

Information and Training: Mandates *training initially* upon assignment and *annually* -- employees who have received appropriate training within the past year need only receive additional training in items not previously covered. Training must include making accessible a copy of the regulatory text of the standard and explanation of its contents, general discussion on bloodborne diseases and their transmission, exposure control plan, engineering and work practice controls, personal protective equipment, hepatitis B vaccine, response to emergencies involving blood, how to handle exposure incidents, the postexposure evaluation and follow-up program, signs/labels/color-coding. There must be *opportunity for questions and answers,* and the *trainer must be knowledgeable* in the subject matter. *Laboratory and production facility workers* must receive *additional specialized initial training.*

Recordkeeping: Calls for medical records to be kept for each employee with occupational exposure for the *duration of employment plus 30 years,* must be *confidential* and must include name and social security number; hepatitis B vaccination status (including dates); results of any examinations, medical testing and follow-up procedures; a copy of the health care professional's written opinion; and a copy of information provided to the health care professional. Training records must be maintained for 3 years and must include dates, contents of the training program or a summary, trainer's name and qualifications, and names and job titles of all persons attending the sessions. Medical records must be made *available to the subject employee,* anyone with written consent of the employee, OSHA, and National Institute for Occupational Safety and Health (NIOSH) -- they are not available to the employer. Disposal of records must be in accord with OSHA's standard covering access to records.

Source: Occupational Safety and Health Administration, 29 CFR Part 1910.1030.

Other Health and Safety Standards

Besides the OSHA regulations regarding bloodborne pathogens and hazard communication, there are other health and safety standards that apply to medical offices, including regulations about air contaminants, fire safety, electrical hazards, etc. Please contact the OSHA office in your state for more information on OSHA standards not addressed in this resource kit.

Medical Waste

Besides the OSHA regulations, each state has regulations regarding medical waste disposal. The types of medical wastes that are regulated include infectious waste, potentially infectious medical waste, untreated infectious waste, medical waste, special waste from health care related facilities, and radioactive materials. In many states, physicians are exempt from these regulations because of the relatively small amounts of waste produced in physicians' offices. However, it is the responsibility of the physician to be familiar with state regulations regarding medical waste management, and respond accordingly. For more information on this topic, please contact the OSHA office in your state.

Report of the Committee on Infectious Diseases

Reprinted from *Report of the Committee on Infectious Diseases,* 23rd edition
Copyright 1994 by the American Academy of Pediatrics

For information on ordering copies of
Report of the Committee on Infectious Diseases, contact:
American Academy of Pediatrics
Division of Publications
141 Northwest Point Blvd, PO Box 927
Elk Grove Village, IL 60009-0927
708/228-5005

AIDS and HIV INFECTIONS

Clinical Manifestations: Human immunodeficiency virus (HIV) infection in children causes a broad spectrum of disease and a varied clinical course. Acquired immunodeficiency syndrome (AIDS) represents the most severe end of the clinical spectrum. The current Centers for Disease Control and Prevention (CDC) surveillance definition for AIDS is given in Table 3.18 (p 255). Patients meeting these criteria for AIDS (see Table 3.18) must be reported to the appropriate public health department. In many states, HIV infection must be reported. The CDC has established a pediatric classification system for children younger than 13 years who are born to HIV-infected mothers or are known to be infected with HIV (see Table 3.19, p 256). This classification is currently being revised (as of December 1993).

The manifestations of HIV infection include generalized lymphadenopthy, hepatomegaly, splenomegaly, failure to thrive, oral candidiasis, recurrent diarrhea, parotitis, cardiomyopathy, hepatitis, nephropathy, central nervous system (CNS) disease (including developmental delay, which can be progressive), lymphoid interstitial pneumonia, recurrent invasive bacterial infections, opportunistic infections, and specified malignancies (Table 3.18, p 255).

Pneumocystis carinii pneumonia (PCP) is the most common, serious opportunistic infection in children with HIV infection, and it is associated with high mortality (see *Pneumocystis carinii Infections*, p 376). Most frequently, PCP occurs in infants between 3 and 12 months of age who acquired infection before or at birth, but it can occur in infants younger than 3 months of age. Other common opportunistic infections in children include *Candida* esophagitis, disseminated cytomegalovirus infection, chronic or disseminated herpes simplex virus infection, *Mycobacterium avium* complex (MAC) infection, chronic enteritis caused by *Cryptosporidium* or other agents, and, less commonly, disseminated or CNS cryptococcal or *Toxoplasma* infection.

Malignancies in pediatric HIV infection have been relatively uncommon to date, but certain lymphomas, including those of the CNS and non-Hodgkin's B-cell lymphomas of the Burkitt type, occur much more frequently in children with HIV infection than in nonimmunocompromised children. Kaposi's sarcoma is very rare in children.

The development of opportunistic infections, particularly PCP, progressive neurologic disease, and severe wasting is associated with a poor prognosis. The prognosis for survival is also poor in children infected perinatally who become symptomatic in the first year of life. With earlier and more effective treatment, survival is likely to improve.

Laboratory findings. The most notable finding, particularly as the disease progresses, is an increasing loss of T-lymphocyte immunity. Initially, the peripheral blood lymphocyte count can be normal, but, eventually, lymphopenia develops because of a decrease in the total number of circulating T-lymphocytes. The cells most affected are the T-helper (CD4) lymphocytes. The T-suppressor (CD8) lymphocytes usually increase in number initially and are not depleted until late in the course of the infection. These changes in cell populations result in a decrease of the normal CD4-to-CD8 cell ratio. This nonspecific finding, although characteristic of HIV infection, also occurs with other acute viral infections, such as those caused by cytomegalovirus or Epstein-Barr virus. The normal values for peripheral CD4 lymphocyte counts and percentages are age related (see Treatment, p 261, including Table 3.20, p 262). Response of T-lymphocytes to plant lectin mitogens (phytohemagglutinin, concanavalin A, and particularly pokeweed) are decreased or absent, and patients may be anergic to skin test antigens such as mumps, *Candida*, *Trichophyton*, tetanus, and tuberculin (Purified Protein Derivative [PPD]).

B-lymphocytes remain normal or are increased in number. Serum immunoglobulin (IG) concentrations, particularly IgG and IgA, are frequently elevated. A few patients will develop panhypogammaglobulinemia. Specific antibody responses to antigens to which the patient has not previously been exposed can be abnormal. Measuring the serum antibody response to measles vaccine administered to children 12 months or older, or to tetanus after three doses of DTP can be useful for assessing humoral responsiveness.

Etiology: AIDS is caused by RNA cytopathic human retroviruses, specifically, human immunodeficiency virus type 1 (HIV-1) and, less commonly, HIV-2, a related virus that is extremely uncommon in the United States but is more common in West Africa. Human immunodeficiency virus is particularly tropic for T-helper (CD4) lymphocytes and other cells such as macrophages that have CD4 receptors. The role of cofactors, such as simultaneous infection with other infectious agents or malnutrition, in the natural history of HIV infection is not known.

Epidemiology: Humans are the only known reservoir of HIV, although related viruses have been

TABLE 3.18—Centers for Disease Control and Prevention Surveillance Case Definition for AIDS—Diagnoses Indicative of AIDS in Children, Adolescents, and Adults [a]

1. **All ages:**
   Candidiasis of the esophagus [b,c]
   Candidiasis of the trachea, bronchi, or lungs [b]
   Coccidioidomycosis, disseminated or extrapulmonary [d]
   Cryptococcosis, extrapulmonary [b]
   Cryptosporidiosis, chronic intestinal [b]
   Cytomegalovirus disease (other than liver, spleen, nodes) onset at >1 month of age [b]
   Cytomegalovirus retinitis (with loss of vision) [b,c]
   Herpes simplex ulcer, chronic (>1 month duration) or pneumonitis or esophagitis onset at >1 month of age [b]
   HIV encephalopathy [d]
   Histoplasmosis, disseminated or extrapulmonary [d]
   Isosporiasis, chronic intestinal (>1 month duration) [d]
   Kaposi's sarcoma [b,c]
   Lymphoma, primary brain [b]
   Lymphoma (Burkitt's, or immunoblastic sarcoma) [d]
   Mycobacterium avium complex or *M kansasii*, disseminated, or extrapulmonary [b]
   M tuberculosis disseminated, or extrapulmonary [d]
   Mycobacterium, other species or unidentified species, disseminated or extrapulmonary [c]
   Pneumocystis carinii pneumonia [b,c]
   Progressive multifocal leukoencephalopathy [b]
   Toxoplasmosis of brain, onset at 1 month of age [b,c]
   Wasting syndrome due to HIV [d]

2. **Additional diagnoses applicable for children <13 years of age:**
   Lymphoid interstitial pneumonitis [b,c]
   Multiple or recurrent serious bacterial infections [d]

3. **Additional diagnoses for adolescents (≥13 years of age) and for adults:**
   Cervical cancer, invasive [d]
   M tuberculosis, pulmonary [d]
   Pneumonia, recurrent [d]
   Salmonella septicemia, recurrent [d]
   CD4 T-lymphocyte count of <200 cells/mm^3 or a CD4 percentage of <14 [d]

---

[a]Adapted from Centers for Disease Control and Prevention. 1993 revised classification system for HIV infection and expanded surveillance case definition for AIDS among adolescents and adults. *MMWR*. 1992;41(RR-17):1-19.

[b]If indicator disease is diagnosed definitively (eg, by biopsy or culture) and no other cause of immunodeficiency is present, laboratory documentation of HIV infection is not required.

[c]Presumptive diagnosis of indicator disease is accepted if laboratory evidence of HIV infection is present.

[d]Laboratory evidence of HIV infection is required.

identified in monkeys. Since retroviruses integrate into the target cell genome as proviruses and the viral genome is copied during cell replication, the virus persists in infected individuals for life. Human immunodeficiency virus has been isolated from blood (including lymphocytes, macrophages, and plasma), other body fluids such as cerebrospinal fluid, pleural fluids, human milk, semen, cervical secretions, saliva, urine, and tears. However, only blood, semen, cervical secretions, and human milk have been implicated epidemiologically in the transmission of infection.

Currently, the predominant modes of HIV transmission in the United States are via (1) sexual contact (both homosexual and heterosexual); (2) percutaneous or mucous membrane exposure to contaminated needles or other sharp instruments; and (3) mother-to-infant transmission before or around the time of birth. Transfusion of blood, blood components, or clotting factor concentrates is now rarely a mode of HIV transmission because of exclusion of infected donors, heat treatment of clotting factor concentrates, and the availability of recombinant clotting factors. In the absence of

TABLE 3.19—Classification System for HIV Infection in Children Younger Than 13 Years*

Class P–O.	Indeterminate Infection. Includes perinatally exposed infants and children younger than 15 months who cannot be classified as definitely infected according to the above definition but who have antibody to HIV, indicating exposure to a mother who is infected.	
Class P–1.	Asymptomatic Infection.	
	Subclass A.	Normal immune function
	Subclass B.	Abnormal immune function
	Subclass C.	Immune function not tested
Class P–2.	Symptomatic Infection.	
	Subclass A.	Nonspecific findings
	Subclass B.	Progressive neurologic disease
	Subclass C.	Lymphoid interstitial pneumonitis
	Subclass D.	Secondary infectious disease
	Category D–1.	Specified secondary infectious diseases listed in the CDC surveillance definition for AIDS
	Category D–2.	Recurrent serious bacterial infections
	Category D–3.	Other specified secondary infectious diseases
	Subclass E.	Secondary cancers
	Category E–1.	Specified secondary cancers listed in the CDC surveillance definition for AIDS
	Category E–2.	Other cancers possibly secondary to HIV infection
	Subclass F.	Other diseases possibly due to HIV infection. Includes children with other conditions possibly due to HIV infection not listed in the above subclasses, such as hepatitis, cardiopathy, nephropathy, hematologic disorders (anemia, thrombocytopenia), and dermatologic diseases.

*From Centers for Disease Control: Classification for human immunodeficiency virus (HIV) infection in children under 13 years of age. *MMWR.* 1987;36:225-230,235-236.

documented parenteral, mucous membrane, or skin contact with blood, transmission of HIV, as of December 1993, has rarely been demonstrated to occur in families or households, in schools or child care settings, or with routine care in hospitals or clinics.

Accidental exposure of health care personnel to HIV, such as from needlestick injuries, has rarely resulted in HIV infection. The risk of infection after a needlestick exposure to HIV-infected blood is approximately 0.3%. Many of the cases that have occurred might have been prevented by careful adherence to infection control measures, especially during emergencies.

AIDS in children and adolescents has accounted for 2% of all reported cases of AIDS in the United States. However, the total number of reported cases in these age groups continues to increase. Acquisition of HIV during adolescence contributes to the large number of AIDS cases in young adults. Adolescent risk factors for HIV infection are similar to those for adults.

Most infected children in the United States have been born to families in which one or both parents have HIV infection. The remainder, including patients with hemophilia or other coagulation disorders, received contaminated blood, its components, or clotting factor concentrates. A few cases of HIV infection in children have resulted from sexual abuse by an HIV-seropositive individual. Less than 5% of cases have been reported to have no identifiable risk factor, and after careful investigation, most are reclassified into one of the established risk factor groups. In some cases, available information is inadequate to determine reclassification.

The risk of infection for an infant born to an HIV-seropositive mother is estimated to be between 13% and 39%. The exact timing of transmission from an infected mother to her infant is uncertain, but evidence suggests that transmission may occur in utero, around the time of delivery, or postpartum through breast-feeding. The available evidence suggests that the majority of infections occur in the perinatal period. Some studies suggest higher rates of perinatal transmission in women with advanced disease, low peripheral CD4 lymphocyte counts, and high viral concentrations as evidenced by HIV p24 antigenemia. Prevention of transmission by cesarean section has not been clearly demonstrated.

Human immunodeficiency virus DNA has been detected in both the cellular and cell-free fractions of human breast milk, and breast-feeding has been implicated in the transmission of HIV infection, especially in mothers who acquired HIV in the postpartum period. These women may have a higher rate of transmission because they, as a result of recent HIV acquisition, have high concentrations of virus. The additional risk of HIV transmission to infants through breast-feeding for women who were infected before pregnancy or early in gestation is uncertain. Data from different populations are inconsistent and analyses are confounded by the different epidemiologic circumstances and study methods in these populations.

The **incubation period** of symptomatic HIV infection (ie, disease) is variable, ranging from months to years. The median age of onset of symptoms is estimated to be 3 years for infants infected perinatally. However, some children exhibit manifestations of infection during the first year of life, whereas others are asymptomatic until they are 5 years or older. In transfusion-associated cases in young children, the median incubation period for onset of clinical disease has been estimated to be 3.5 years, but with considerable individual variability. Other than infants born of infected mothers, persons infected with HIV usually develop serum antibody to HIV within 6 to 12 weeks after infection.

Diagnostic Tests: Diagnosis of HIV infection is usually made by serum antibody tests except in children younger than 18 months of age in whom passively acquired maternal antibody may be present.

Enzyme immunoassays (EIA) are most widely used to screen for HIV antibody. These tests are highly sensitive and specific, but false-positive results occur in a small percentage of cases. Repeat EIA testing of initially reactive specimens is required to reduce the likelihood of laboratory error; repeatedly reactive tests are highly reliable. Western blot or immunofluorescent antibody tests should be used for confirmation. A positive HIV antibody test in a child 18 months of age or older is usually indicative of infection.

Serum antibodies to HIV are present in almost all infected persons, although some patients with AIDS become seronegative late in disease. Some children with HIV infection may test negative for HIV antibody because they have hypogammaglobulinemia, or late in disease may be unable to produce antibody. Rarely, an HIV-infected child is antibody negative by EIA testing but positive on Western blot or positive by other virologic tests, such as culture or polymerase chain reaction (PCR).

Infants born to HIV-seropositive women pose a special diagnostic challenge since these infants are almost always seropositive at birth as the result of transplacental acquisition of maternal antibody, whether or not they are infected, and these serum antibodies can be detectable in the infant for as long as 18 months after birth. Thus, IgG antibody tests for HIV are not useful for diagnosis in the child younger than 18 months of age. However, the diagnosis can be made in infants in the first few months of life by other tests, specifically, positive HIV culture, detection of HIV DNA sequences using the PCR, detection of IgA-specific anti-HIV antibodies (after 3 months of age), and positive HIV-p24 antigen assay after acid dissociation. One or more of these tests are generally available at referral centers caring for HIV-infected children.

Using these assays, most infected infants can be diagnosed by 3 to 6 months of age. For an infant born to an HIV-seropositive mother, an initial diagnostic assay should be performed by approximately 1 month of age or as soon as possible thereafter. If the assay is negative, repeat testing between 3 and 6 months of age is indicated. A positive HIV culture, PCR and/or p24 antigen detection assay constitutes presumptive evidence of HIV infection, and a second diagnostic test should be subsequently performed, using either the same assay or one of the other two assays, to confirm the diagnosis. If an infant younger than 18 months of age who has a positive serologic test for HIV develops an AIDS-defining illness (see Table 3.18, p 255), the diagnosis of HIV infection is established even if virologic tests are negative.

The child who has negative virologic tests at 6 months of age requires continued serologic follow-up to document disappearance of maternal HIV antibody. An infant born to a seropositive mother who is HIV antibody negative at two consecutive times by 18 months of age, has normal immune function studies, and never has had a positive virologic test (culture, PCR, or p24 antigen) for HIV is a seroreverter and should be considered not to be infected. Despite two or more negative serologic tests, the National Pediatric HIV Resource Center recommends a final test at 24 months of age to decrease the possibility of misdiagnosing an infected, but antibody- negative child.*

Since interpretation of the available diagnostic tests may be complex, the pediatrician should consult with an HIV specialist to assist in the interpretation of diagnostic assays.

Perinatal HIV Serologic Testing. Recommendations of the AAP Task Force on Pediatric AIDS include the following[†]:

- HIV testing should be routinely offered to all pregnant women and women of childbearing age throughout the United States.
- HIV testing should be routinely recommended and encouraged for all pregnant women and women of childbearing age at increased risk of HIV infection because of high-risk behaviors or because they live in areas (eg, state, metropolitan area, or city) with an HIV seroprevalence rate among pregnant women and newborns of 1:1,000 or more.
- Newborn testing should be routinely recommended and encouraged in mothers with known high-risk behaviors or from high-seroprevalence areas who have not been tested.
- HIV testing should be recommended and encouraged for abandoned infants and for infants otherwise in need of foster or adoptive care, as needed to facilitate placement and care. Courts should adopt methods for rapid processing of court orders to allow HIV testing of abandoned infants or those in foster care when follow-up adoption or initial placement may be facilitated by such testing.
- Testing in the perinatal period should be determined by specified policies that ensure retesting, education, informed consent, counseling, and follow-up criteria.

- Anonymous seroprevalence surveys should be continued and expanded to provide ongoing information on HIV seroprevalence in specific metropolitan areas and states. These surveys are not a substitute for individual counseling and testing, but they provide important public health information.
- Pediatricians or other primary pediatric caregivers should be informed whenever an infant is born to a known HIV-seropositive mother so that appropriate care and follow-up testing can be undertaken.
- Development of testing programs without addressing access to care is inappropriate. However, testing programs that may benefit the mother, fetus, and newborn cannot be delayed until access problems have been resolved completely.
- The Academy opposes mandatory (involuntary) maternal and/or newborn testing at this time.

Informed Consent for HIV Serologic Testing. Testing for HIV infection is unlike most routine blood testing in that substantial psychosocial risks can be incurred. When testing an infant or child, parents or other primary caretakers, and patients, if old enough to comprehend, should be counseled about the possible risks and benefits of testing and the consequences of HIV infection. Oral consent should be obtained from the parent or legal guardian and recorded in the patient's chart. Special written consent procedures for HIV testing should be discouraged as they can inhibit the performance of testing without adding significant benefit. Nevertheless, state and local laws and hospital regulations should be considered in deciding whether written consent is required. The necessity for counseling and consent should not deter efforts to undertake appropriate diagnostic testing for HIV infection. Refusal to give consent does not relieve the physician of the professional and legal responsibilities to their patients. If the physician believes that testing is essential to the child's health, authorization for testing will need to be obtained by other means. The results of serologic tests should be discussed in person with the family, primary caretaker, and, if appropriate according to age, the patient; if positive, appropriate counseling and subsequent follow-up care must be provided. Maintaining confidentiality in all cases is essential to preserving patient and parent trust and consent.

Treatment: Primary care physicians are encouraged to actively participate in the care of HIV-infected patients.

---

*Working Group on Antiretroviral Therapy: National Pediatric HIV Resource Center. Antiretroviral therapy and medical management of the human immunodeficiency virus-infected child. *Pediatr Infect Dis J.* 1993;12:513-522

[†]For further information, see Task Force on Pediatric AIDS. Perinatal human immunodeficiency virus (HIV) testing. *Pediatrics.* 1992;89:791-794

Antiretroviral therapy has become a standard of care for all children with symptomatic HIV infection. Guidelines for the institution of antiretroviral therapy in infants and children with HIV infection have been formulated by the Working Group on Antiretroviral Therapy convened by the National Pediatric HIV Resource Center.[*] The clinical and immunologic criteria for initiating therapy are listed in Table 3.20 (p 262). Current data are insufficient to recommend therapy in asymptomatic children with normal age-adjusted CD4 lymphocyte counts, including those with normal physical examinations as well as those with only lymphadenopathy, hepatomegaly, or hypergammaglobulinemia.

Oral zidovudine has been approved for use in children as well as in adolescents and adults. It is recommended for HIV-infected adults and adolescents with symptomatic HIV infection and often for those with CD4 lymphocyte counts of less than 500/mm^3. For children 4 weeks of age or older with symptomatic HIV infection or immunosuppression (see Table 3.20, p 262), zidovudine is also recommended as initial therapy and is generally well tolerated. For dosage recommendations, see Antiviral Drugs, p 567. The most common side effect is hematologic toxicity (anemia and/or neutropenia). Hence, complete blood and platelet counts should be monitored monthly during therapy.

Changes in antiretroviral therapy should be made in consultation with a specialist experienced in the management of HIV infection, especially since therapeutic alternatives are limited. Disease progression in children is usually defined as deterioration of CNS function or growth failure. Other evidence of disease progression can include development of a new AIDS-defining opportunistic infection (Table 3.18, p 255), symptomatic HIV-associated cardiomyopathy, nephrotic syndrome, or significant, otherwise unexplained serum transaminase elevations (more than five times normal). Laboratory criteria for disease progression mandating a change in drug therapy are not clearly defined in children, particularly in the absence of clinical progression.

Didanosine (DDI), formerly termed dideoxyinosine, is an alternative therapy for children who cannot tolerate zidovudine or whose disease has progressed while receiving zidovudine therapy. For dosage recommendations, see Antiviral Drugs (p 567).

For optimal absorption of DDI, adequate buffering of stomach acid is necessary, and no food or drink should be taken for at least 30 minutes before and after drug administration. Side effects include pancreatitis and peripheral retinal depigmentation without associated visual impairment. Peripheral neuropathy has been reported in adults but not in children receiving the commonly used doses. Monthly monitoring of complete blood counts and of the serum amylase, or whenever abdominal symptoms occur, is essential.

Zalcitabine (DDC) has recently been approved for use in adults, but it is not yet approved for use in children. It is indicated for use in combination with zidovudine for adults with symptomatic HIV infection or CD4 lymphocyte counts equal to or less than 300/mm^3. Multicenter clinical trials are evaluating drug combinations, including zidovudine with DDI, and zidovudine with DDC, in children.

Other new antiretroviral drugs, immunomodulators, and vaccines for therapeutic use are under evaluation. Further information on therapeutic trials in HIV-infected children can be obtained from the Pediatric Clinical Trials Group, Pediatric Branch, National Cancer Institute (see Directory of Telephone Numbers, p 601).

The value of intravenous immune globulin (IGIV) in children with HIV infection has been evaluated in several trials. The Working Group on Antiretroviral Therapy has recommended routine IGIV therapy in combination with an antiviral agent for children with humoral immunodeficiency including (1) hypogammaglobulinemia (IgG less than 250 mg/mL); (2) recurrent, serious bacterial infections (defined as two or more serious bacterial infections such as bacteremia, meningitis, or pneumonia in a 1-year period); (3) children who fail to form antibodies to common antigens; and (4) children living in areas where measles is highly prevalent who have not developed an antibody response after two doses (1 month or more apart) of MMR.[†] The dose of IGIV is 400 mg/kg per dose given every 4 weeks. Intravenous immune globulin may also be useful in the treatment of HIV-associated thrombocytopenia at a dose of 500 to 1,000 mg/kg/d for 3 to 5 days. In addition, children with bronchiectasis despite treatment with the standard medical regimen of cyclic antibiotics and aggressive respiratory therapy might benefit from adjunctive IGIV therapy at 600 mg/kg per dose, given monthly.

---

[*]For detailed, further information, see Working Group on Antiretroviral Therapy: National Pediatric HIV Resource Center. Antiretroviral therapy and medical management of the human immunodeficiency virus-infected child. *Pediatr Infect Dis J*. 1993;12:513-522

[†]Working Group on Antiretroviral Therapy: National Pediatric HIV Resource Center. Antiretroviral therapy and medical management of the human immunodeficiency virus-infected child. *Pediatr Infect Dis J*. 1993;12:513-522.

TABLE 3.20—Recommendations for Use of Antiretroviral Therapy in Infants and Children With Proven HIV Infection*

- The presence of any of the HIV-associated clinical conditions listed below warrants initiation of antiretroviral therapy, independent of CD4 lymphocyte count:

    a. AIDS-defining opportunistic infection
    b. Wasting disease (crossing two percentiles over time)
    c. Failure to thrive (below the 5th percentile for age and falling from the growth curve)
    d. Progressive encephalopathy
    e. Malignancy
    f. Recurrent septicemia/meningitis
    g. Thrombocytopenia <75,000 platelets/mm^3
    h. Hypogammaglobulinemia (total IgG/IgM/IgA <250 mg/mL)

- If CD4 lymphocyte counts are less than the following age-adjusted concentrations, therapy should be initiated independent of clinical findings:

    CD4 absolute count

    <1,750 cells/mm^3 for children younger than 1 y
    <1,000 cells/mm^3 for children 1-2 y
    <750 cells/mm^3 for children 2-6 y
    <500 cells/mm^3 for children older than 6 y

    CD4 percentage (of the total peripheral lymphocyte count)

    <30% for children younger than 1 y
    <25% for children 1-2 y
    <20% for children older than 2 y

- Therapy should also be considered in children with the following clinical conditions, even if occurring as an isolated finding, independent of the CD4 lymphocyte count:

    Lymphoid interstitial pneumonitis
    Parotitis
    Splenomegaly
    Persistent oral candidiasis
    Recurrent and/or chronic diarrhea
    Cardiomyopathy
    Nephropathy
    Hepatitis
    Endocrinopathy
    Recurrent and/or chronic bacterial infections, such as sinusitis/pneumonia
    Recurrent herpes simplex and/or varicella-zoster infections
    Neutropenia (<750 neutrophils/mm^3)
    Anemia
    Neurodevelopmental abnormalities

---

*For further information, see Working Group on Antiretroviral Therapy: National Pediatric HIV Resource Center. Antiretroviral therapy and medical management of the human immunodeficiency virus-infected child. *Pediatr Infect Dis J*. 1993;12:513-522.

Early diagnosis and aggressive treatment of opportunistic infections may prolong survival. Since PCP can be an early complication of perinatally acquired HIV infection and mortality is high, chemoprophylaxis should be given to HIV-infected children at risk for PCP. For further information, see *Pneumocystis carinii* Infections, p 377.

Chemoprophylaxis may also be warranted for MAC infections (see Diseases Caused by Nontuberculous Mycobacteria, p 503).

Immunization Recommendations (see also Table 3.21, p 264).

Children With Symptomatic HIV Infection. In general, live-virus (eg, oral poliovirus) vaccines and live-bacterial (eg, bacillus Calmette-Guerin) vaccines should not be given to patients with AIDS or other clinical manifestations of HIV infection who are immunosuppressed. Measles, mumps, and rubella (MMR) vaccine combined is an exception. For routine immunizations, DTP, hepatitis B, *Haemophilus influenzae* type b conjugate, inactivated poliovirus (IPV), and MMR vaccines should be given according to the usual immunization schedule (see Tables 1.3 and 1.4, pp 23 and 24). Pneumococcal vaccine at 2 years of age and yearly influenza vaccination beginning at age 6 months are also recommended.

The occurrence of severe measles in symptomatic HIV-infected children and the lack of reported serious or unusual reactions to immunization with MMR vaccine have led to the recommendation for measles immunization of HIV-infected children, regardless of symptoms, with MMR vaccine. Although MMR is usually given at 12 to 15 months, if the risk of exposure to measles is increased, such as during an outbreak, these children should receive vaccine at a younger age (see Measles, p 312).

In general, children with symptomatic HIV infection have poor immunologic responses to vaccines. Hence, such children, when exposed to a vaccine-preventable disease such as measles or tetanus, should be considered susceptible regardless of the history of vaccination, and should receive, if indicated, passive immunoprophylaxis (see Passive Immunization of Children With HIV Infection, p 265).

Children With Asymptomatic HIV Infection. Children with asymptomatic HIV infection should receive DTP, IPV, *Haemophilus influenzae* type b conjugate, hepatitis B, IPV, and MMR vaccines, according to the usual immunization schedules (see Tables 1.3 and 1.4, pp 23 and 24). Although oral poliovirus vaccine (OPV) has been given to

these patients without adverse effect, IPV is recommended because both the child and family members may be immunosuppressed as the result of HIV infection and, therefore, may be at risk for vaccine-associated paralytic poliomyelitis caused by vaccine virus infection.

Pneumococcal vaccination is indicated for HIV-infected children 2 years and older in view of their high incidence of invasive pneumococcal infection. Yearly influenza vaccination should be considered for children 6 months or older.

In areas of low tuberculosis prevalence, BCG vaccine is not recommended. However, in areas where the prevalence of tuberculosis is high, the World Health Organization recommends that BCG should be given to all infants at birth, regardless of maternal HIV infection, if the infants are asymptomatic.

Seronegative Children Residing in the Household of a Patient With Symptomatic HIV Infection. In a household with an adult or child immunocompromised as the result of HIV infection, seronegative as well as seropositive children should receive IPV vaccine because the live polioviruses in OPV can be excreted and transmitted to immunosuppressed contacts. MMR vaccine may be given because MMR vaccine viruses are not transmitted. To reduce the risk of transmission of influenza to patients with symptomatic HIV infection, yearly influenza vaccination is indicated for their household contacts (see Influenza, p 280).

Passive Immunization of Children With HIV Infection.

1. *Measles* (see Measles, p 311).
   - Symptomatic HIV-infected children who are exposed to measles should receive immune globulin (IG) prophylaxis (0.5 mL/kg, maximum 15 mL), regardless of vaccination status.
   - Exposed, asymptomatic HIV-infected patients who are susceptible should also receive IG; the recommended dose is 0.25 mL/kg.
   - Children who have received IGIV within 3 weeks of exposure do not require additional passive immunization.
2. *Tetanus.* In the management of wounds classified as tetanus prone (see Tetanus, p 460 and Table 3.45, p 461), children with HIV infection should receive Tetanus Immune Globulin (Human) (TIG) regardless of vaccination status.
3. *Varicella.* Children infected with HIV who are exposed to varicella or zoster and who are susceptible should receive Varicella-Zoster

TABLE 3.21—Recommendations for Routine Immunization of HIV-Infected Children in the United States*

Vaccine†	Known Asymptomatic HIV Infection	Symptomatic HIV Infection
Hepatitis B	Yes	Yes
DTP	Yes	Yes
OPV	No	No
IPV	Yes	Yes
MMR	Yes	Yes
Hib	Yes	Yes
Pneumococcal	Yes	Yes
Influenza	Should be considered	Yes

*See Table 1.3 (p 23) for age at which specific vaccines are indicated.

†DTP = diphtheria and tetanus toxoids and pertussis vaccine; OPV = oral poliovirus vaccine; IPV = inactivated poliovirus vaccine; MMR = live-virus measles, mumps, and rubella; Hib = *Haemophilus influenzae* type b conjugate.

Immune Globulin (VZIG) (see Varicella-Zoster Infections, p 516). Children who have received IGIV or VZIG within 3 weeks of exposure do not require additional passive immunization.

Isolation of the Hospitalized Patient: Universal blood and body fluid precautions should be scrupulously followed by all hospital personnel (see Isolation Precautions, p 92). The risk to health care personnel of acquiring HIV infection from a patient is minimal, even after accidental exposure from a needlestick injury. Nevertheless, every effort should be made to avoid exposures to blood and other body fluids that could contain HIV (see Table 2.4, p 94).

Control Measures:

*Adolescent Education.** Adolescents at risk for HIV infection should have access to HIV testing and knowledge of their serostatus. Attention to the need for informed consent for either testing or the release of information regarding serostatus is crucial. Decisions regarding the disclosure of HIV status to a sexual partner without the consent of the patient should be based on several factors, including whether the partner has a reasonable cause to suspect the risk and take precautions without specific warning; the likelihood the partner is in fact at risk; relevant law that might prohibit or require such disclosure; and the possible effects of such disclosure upon future patients.

Specific recommendations of the AAP Task Force on Pediatric AIDS for pediatricians caring for adolescents are as follows:

- Information regarding HIV infection and AIDS should be regarded as an important component of the anticipatory guidance provided by pediatricians to their adolescent patients. This guidance should include information about transmission, implications of infection, and strategies for prevention including abstinence from behaviors that place adolescents at risk and safer sex practices for those who opt to be sexually active.
- Young persons at risk for HIV infection should be offered diagnostic testing in addition to other educational and counseling services.
- Parental involvement in adolescent health care is a desirable goal. However, the consent of the adolescent alone should be sufficient to provide evaluation and treatment for suspected or confirmed HIV infection.
- The maintenance of confidentiality regarding HIV status is of great importance. Respecting this confidentiality, the pediatrician should use all reasonable means to persuade an infected adolescent to inform his or her sexual partner on a voluntary basis. Involuntary disclosure is a complex question that should be decided on the basis of local law, the relationship between the physician and the patient, the relationship of the physician to the partner, and the degree of perceived risk to the unsuspecting sexual partner.

If adolescents are sexually active, they should be counseled about the correct and consistent use of condoms to reduce the risk of infection (see Sexually Transmitted Diseases, p 103).

School Attendance and Education of Children With HIV Infection. In the absence of blood exposure, HIV infection is not acquired through the types

*For further information, see Task Force on Pediatric AIDS. Adolescents and human immunodeficiency virus infection: the role of the pediatrician in prevention and intervention. *Pediatrics*. 1993;92:626-630.

of contact that usually occur in a school setting, including contact with saliva or tears. Hence, children with HIV infection should not be excluded from school for the protection of other children or personnel. Specific recommendations concerning school attendance of children and adolescents with HIV infection are the following:

- Most school-aged children and adolescents infected with HIV should be allowed to attend school without restrictions, provided the child's physician gives approval.
- The need for a more restricted school environment for some infected children should be evaluated on a case-by-case basis considering conditions that may pose an increased risk to others, such as aggressive biting behavior or the presence of exudative, weeping skin lesions that cannot be covered.
- No one besides the child's parents, other guardians, and physician has an absolute need to know that the child is HIV-infected. The number of personnel aware of the child's condition should be kept to the minimum needed to ensure proper care of the child. The family has the right to inform the school. Persons involved in the care and education of an infected student must respect the student's right to privacy.
- All schools should adopt routine procedures for handling blood or blood-contaminated fluids, including the disposal of sanitary napkins, regardless of whether students with HIV infection are known to be in attendance. School health care workers, teachers, administrators, and other employees should be educated about procedures (see Housekeeping Procedures for Blood and Body Fluids, p 268).
- Children infected with HIV develop progressive immunodeficiency, which increases their risk of experiencing severe complications from infections such as varicella, tuberculosis, measles, cytomegalovirus, and herpes simplex virus. The child's physician should regularly assess the risk of an unrestricted environment on the health of the HIV-infected student, including evaluation of possible contagious diseases in the school (eg, measles, varicella, tuberculosis).
- Routine screening of schoolchildren for HIV infection is not recommended.

As the incidence of HIV infection in children increases, the school population of children with this disease will increase. With the advent of new drug therapy, these children will likely have longer sur-

vival, resulting in an increasing number of HIV-infected children entering school. An understanding of the effect of chronic illness and the recognition of neurodevelopmental problems in these children is essential to provide appropriate educational programs. The AAP Task Force on Pediatric AIDS has made the following recommendations regarding the education of children with HIV infection[*]:

- All children with HIV infection should receive an appropriate education that is adapted to their evolving special needs. The spectrum of needs differs with the stage of the disease.
- HIV infection should be treated like other chronic illnesses that require special education and other related services.
- Continuity of education must be assured whether at school or at home.
- Because of the stigmatization that still exists with this disease, maintaining confidentiality is essential. Disclosures of information should be only with the informed consent of the parents or legal guardians and age-appropriate assent of the student.

Child Care[†] and Foster Care. Current AAP recommendations are as follows[‡]:

- No reason exists to restrict foster care or adoptive placement of children who have HIV infection to protect the health of other family members. The risk of transmission of HIV infection in family environments is negligible.
- No need exists to restrict the placement of HIV-infected children in child care settings to protect personnel or other children because the risk of transmission of HIV in these settings is negligible.
- Child care personnel need not be informed of the HIV status of a child to protect the health of caregivers or other children in the child care environment. In some jurisdictions the child's diagnosis cannot be divulged without the written consent of the parent or legal guardian. Parents may choose to inform the child care provider of the child's diagnosis to support a request that the caregiver observe the child closely for signs of

---

[*]For further information, see Task Force on Pediatric AIDS. Education of children with human immunodeficiency virus infection. *Pediatrics.* 1991;88:645-648.

[†]For additional discussion of recommendations for child care, see Children in Out-of-Home Child Care, p 89.

[‡]Adapted from American Academy of Pediatrics Task Force on Pediatric AIDS. Guidelines for human immunodeficiency virus (HIV)-infected children and their families. *Pediatrics.* 1992;89: 681-683.

illness that might require medical attention and assist the parents with the child's special emotional and social needs.

- Recommended universal precautions should be followed in all child care settings when blood or bloody fluids are being handled, to minimize the possibility of transmission of any blood-borne disease (see Housekeeping Procedures for Blood and Body Fluids, below).
- All preschool child care programs should routinely inform all families whenever a highly infectious illness, such as measles or chickenpox, occurs in any child in that setting. This process will help families protect their immunodeficient children.
- To facilitate foster care or adoptive placement, courts should adopt methods for rapid processing of court orders to allow HIV testing of infants and young children whenever such testing would promote placement. Placement would be promoted most clearly when such court-ordered testing is pursued in areas of high seroprevalence or when the child comes from a high-risk setting.

Adults With HIV Infection Working in Child Care or Schools. Asymptomatic HIV-infected adults may care for children in school or child care settings provided that they do not have exudative skin lesions or other conditions that would allow contact with their body fluids. No data indicate that HIV-infected adults have transmitted HIV in the course of normal child care or school responsibilities.

Adults with symptomatic HIV infection are immunocompromised and at increased risk from infectious diseases of young children. They should consult their physicians regarding the safety of their continuing work.

Housekeeping Procedures for Blood and Body Fluids. In general, routine housekeeping procedures using a commercially available cleaner (detergents, disinfectant-detergents, or chemical germicides) compatible with most surfaces are satisfactory for cleaning spills of vomitus, urine, and feces. Nasal secretions can be removed with tissues and discarded in routine waste containers. For spills involving blood or other body fluids: organic material should be removed, then the surface disinfected with diluted bleach (ie, 1:10 to 1:100). A 1:64 dilution is 1/4 cup bleach diluted in 1 gallon of water. Reusable rubber gloves may be useful for cleaning large spills to avoid contamination of the hands of the person cleaning the spill, but gloves are not essential for cleaning small amounts of blood that can be contained easily by the material used for clean-

ing. Persons involved in cleaning contaminated surfaces should avoid exposure of open skin lesions or mucous membranes to blood or bloody fluids. Whenever possible, disposable towels or tissues should be used and properly discarded, and mops should be rinsed in the disinfectant.

Management and Counseling of Families. Infection acquired by children before or during birth is a disease of the family. Serologic screening of siblings and parents is recommended. In each case, the physician needs to provide education and ongoing counseling regarding HIV and its transmission, and to outline precautions to be taken within the household and the community to prevent spread of this virus.

Infected women need to be made aware of the risk of having an infected child if they become pregnant, and they should be referred for family planning counseling. Infected individuals should not donate blood, plasma, sperm, organs, corneas, bone, other tissues, or breast milk.

The infected child should be taught good hygiene and behavior. How much he or she is told about the illness will depend on age and maturity. Older children and adolescents should be made aware that the disease can be transmitted sexually, and they should be provided with appropriate counseling. Most families are not willing to share the diagnosis with others, since it can create social isolation. Feelings of guilt are common. Family members, including children, can become clinically depressed and require psychiatric counseling.

Breast-feeding (see also Human Milk, p 73). The risk of HIV transmission by breast-feeding, especially from mothers who acquire HIV infection during the postpartum period, has been reported in some studies to be increased. In the United States, where safe, alternative, effective sources of feeding are readily available and affordable, an HIV-infected woman should be counseled not to breast-feed her infant or donate to milk banks. The World Health Organization has recommended that mothers residing in areas where infectious disease and malnutrition are an important cause of mortality early in life should be advised to breast-feed their infants regardless of the mother's HIV serologic status.

Sexual Abuse. After sexual abuse by a person with or at risk for HIV infection, the child should be tested at the time of abuse and at 3 and 6 months after sexual contact for antibodies to HIV (see Sexual Abuse, p 110). If feasible, serologic evaluation of the abuser for HIV infection should be obtained. Counseling of the child and family needs to be provided.

Blood, Blood Components, and Clotting Factors.
Screening blood and plasma for HIV antibody has
dramatically reduced the risk of infection through
transfusion. Nevertheless, careful scrutiny of the
requirements of each patient for blood, its components, or clotting factors is important.

Transmission of HIV through contaminated
clotting-factor concentrates has been virtually eliminated in the United States. All plasma-derived factor
VIII and factor IX concentrates available in the United
States are now manufactured from plasma screened
for HIV antibody. Additionally, the concentrates are
treated with heat, solvents, or detergents for inactiva-
tion of HIV (as well as other agents including hepatitis
B and hepatitis C viruses). Some concentrates
also undergo monoclonal antibody purification.
Cryoprecipitate from single or pooled donor plasma
is screened for anti-HIV antibody but does not undergo any process to inactivate HIV or other viruses.
Patients with hemophilia should be managed in
consultation with specialists familiar with current
aspects of treatment, such as desmopressin for the
treatment of individuals with mild or moderate
factor VIII deficiency. Recombinant factor replace-
ment is now available.

Exposed Health Care Workers.[*] Management of
the health care worker who has had a percutaneous or
mucous membrane exposure to blood or bloody secretions from an HIV-positive patient should include the
following:

1. Confirmation that the patient is HIV positive.
2. Evaluation of the health care worker clinically
   and serologically for evidence of HIV infection
   as soon as possible after the exposure. If the
   health care worker is seronegative, he or she
   should be retested at 6 weeks, 3 months, and
   6 months after exposure to determine whether
   transmission has occurred. Most exposed individuals who have been infected will serocon-
   vert during the first 12 weeks after exposure.
3. Immediately informing the exposed health
   care worker of the availability of zidovudine
   for chemoprophylaxis. The data on the use of
   zidovudine for postexposure prophylaxis,
   however, are inadequate to establish its efficacy
   or safety. In the absence of conclusive data,
   many medical centers have adopted a protocol
   for offering zidovudine chemoprophylaxis after
   occupational exposures. If given, zidovudine
   should be started as soon as possible after
   exposure at a dose (for adults) of 200 mg
   every 4 hours for 4 to 6 weeks.
4. Counseling about the risks from the exposure
   and possible benefits of zidovudine.

---

[*]For additional information, see Centers for Disease Control. Guidelines
for prevention of transmission of human immunodeficiency virus and hepatitis B virus to health-care and public-safety workers. *MMWR*. 1989;38
(5-6):9-10.

School Health: Policy and Practice

Reprinted from *School Health: Policy and Practice, 5th edition*
Copyright 1993 by the American Academy of Pediatrics

For information on ordering copies of
School Health: Policy and Practice, contact:
American Academy of Pediatrics
Division of Publications
141 Northwest Point Blvd, PO Box 927
Elk Grove Village, IL 60009-0927
800/433-9016

HIV — STUDENTS AND SCHOOL PERSONNEL

The human immunodeficiency virus (HIV) epidemic has been with us since cases of HIV infection first were reported in 1980. Treatment regimens are available, but treatment is not yet fully effective. Because the HIV virus is transmitted almost exclusively by sexual behavior that adolescents and adults can alter, educational programs could be effective in the prevention of the spread of HIV infection. Children with HIV infection most likely have acquired it at birth or from a transfusion of contaminated blood products.

Children with HIV infection can participate in all activities in school to the extent that their health permits. They should not be excluded from school, nor should they be isolated within the school setting.

Epidemiology

Acquired immunodeficiency syndrome (AIDS) is a major leading cause of death among children 1 to 4 years of age and in young people between the ages of 15 and 24. As of July 1992, there were 222,419 cases of reported AIDS in the United States. Of these cases, 3,694 were infants and children under the age of 13, and 854 were adolescents through age 19 (630 males and 224 females). For every child who actually has AIDS, it is estimated that 2 to 10 children are infected with the HIV virus. By 1995, 5.7 million people will be infected with HIV in the United States. A total of $10 billion will be expended for treatment of people infected by HIV. That figure will jump to $15 billion annually in the mid-1990s. New York state has the highest incidence of AIDS in patients under the age of 13, with 1,043 cases of which 940 were in New York City. This is followed by Florida (588), New Jersey (378), California (241), and Puerto Rico (200).

Although HIV has been found in blood; saliva; urine; cervical secretion; cerebral, spinal, and pleural fluid; and human milk, transmission of the virus has only occurred through blood, semen, cervical secretions, and, sometimes, through breast milk. Transmission from an infected person to an uninfected person has occurred by only three major routes: sexual intercourse, inoculation of blood (ie, drug users who share syringes and needles for injections), and blood transfusion from an infected source. Congenital or perinatal transmission from a woman to her fetus or newborn accounts for the majority of infants and children with HIV infections. Due in part to the unusually long latency period between the onset of

HIV infection and the appearance of symptoms, HIV infection among adolescents may be much greater than the apparent low incidence of AIDS cases in adolescents. There is every indication that HIV infection can spread, and is spreading, to all segments of our society.

The HIV infection has a devastating impact on children and their families, schools, and communities. Handicaps resulting from the disease can cause social and psychological problems. Myths circulate that the disease can be transmitted by casual contact. This causes fear and anxiety and results in discrimination. Increasing costs for AIDS patients threaten to absorb a disproportionate amount of health care funds, thus placing other valuable social welfare resources and needs in competition with HIV-related services. A collaborative approach will be needed.

Children with HIV infection can be admitted freely to all schools to the extent to which their health will permit. This places a great burden on special services, however, and confidentiality problems ensue involving the patient's right-to-privacy versus the school's right-to-know. Related services may need to be utilized without the school knowing the true diagnosis.

Children with HIV infections show evidence of increasing cognitive dysfunction resulting in a higher incidence of learning disabilities and school problems. These children may progress to a need for home instruction as well as occupational and physical therapy similar to that needed to treat cerebral palsy. Behavioral problems also occur involving depression, anxiety, family disruption, and hostility, resulting in the need for increasing mental health services.

Prevention offers the chief means of decreasing the incidence of HIV infection. Thorough screening methods have practically eliminated infected blood transfusions as a source of HIV. Use of condoms together with virucidal vaginal gels can prevent HIV infection during intercourse. Sterile needle exchange programs for drug abusers combined with treatment programs have been proposed to reduce this particular source of HIV infection. Many authorities believe that these are the most effective ways to prevent HIV infections. Voluntary neonatal screening programs together with counseling will help us to track and treat newborn HIV infections. The most effective and universally accepted method of HIV prevention is education done in an organized, comprehensive, well-developed manner by a coalition of schools and the community. The pediatrician can play a pivotal role in implementing these efforts and acting as a case manager when required.

AIDS Education as a Major Prevention of Transmission

Educational programs can be effective in the prevention of the spread of HIV infection. In October 1986, Surgeon General C. Everett Koop, MD, issued a report on AIDS in which he stated: "AIDS education should start in early elementary school and in the home so the children could grow up knowing the behavior to avoid in order to protect themselves." The Office of School Health and Education Projects at the Centers for Disease Control (CDC) in 1986 convened a special task force in order to write guidelines for effective school health education to prevent the spread of AIDS.

These guidelines state that:
1. Education about AIDS would be most appropriate and effective when carried out within a comprehensive school health program; that State Departments of Education and Health should work together in order to establish this; that community involvement was essential; and that programs should be developed also to address the developmental needs of students in school and out-of-school youth and minorities.
2. Programs should be taught by qualified teachers.
3. Young people should abstain from sexual intercourse until ready to establish a mutually monogamous relationship.
4. Students should refrain from using illicit drugs and avoid sharing needles.
5. If abstinence cannot be practiced, then a latex condom should be used with a virucidal spermicide.
6. Students should seek counseling and testing when HIV infection is suspected.

These guidelines also contain specific suggestions as to the content of AIDS education. In early elementary school, AIDS education should be designed to allay excessive fears of the epidemic and discuss the difference between sickness and health. In late elementary school, the concept of viral infection and the nature of AIDS can be discussed. In junior and senior high school, the specifics of the sexual transmission of AIDS and prevention, discrimination,

civil rights issues, and other social aspects should be discussed. The report also suggests that sufficient curriculum time and resources be allotted at each grade level to ensure that the student acquire essential knowledge and that the criteria for program assessment be provided. The report was delayed for over a year due to governmental concerns about its content, but it finally was released and published in *Morbidity Mortality Weekly Report* in January 1988.

In September 1987, the CDC had awarded funds totalling $6 million for underwriting a number of model education programs. Funds for training and developmental grants were awarded to national educational organizations and groups serving minorities and out-of-school youth, to the state and local educational agencies in areas with a high incidence of AIDS, and to private curriculum development organizations. As a result of these efforts, a number of organizations established effective AIDS education programs. Included among these were the American School Health Association, the National Education Association, and the American Association of Superintendents and Administrators. These organizations sought consultation with the American Academy of Pediatrics in order to help develop their programs. The CDC also established a combined health information data base in order to provide information about AIDS education programs to organizations wishing to develop programs. Organizations or individuals can contact the data base and obtain information regarding programs registered with the CDC. Further information about these programs can be obtained by written request from the Division of Adolescent and School Health.* Additional information about AIDS education programs is also provided in this chapter.

Policies

Hysteria and fear were encountered when efforts were made to admit children with HIV infections to public schools. In many states and school systems, children were put in special self-contained classrooms or educated at home. The CDC and the American Academy of Pediatrics have issued statements stating that children with HIV infection can attend school. Both the CDC and the American Academy of Pediatrics now believe that children with HIV infection can attend school in an unrestricted manner and do not need to be isolated within the classroom, either for the protection of other chil-

---

*Division of Adolescent and School Health, Mail Stop K-31, 4770 Buford Highway NE, Atlanta, GA 30341,-3724.

dren or for their own protection. School district policies should reflect these official policies.

Confidentiality

Confidentiality is the keystone to ensuring the education of the child with HIV. The school's request for information needed to educate the child must be balanced by the need to safeguard the rights of the patient. The primary role of the pediatrician is to represent the patient and the family. Although the school environment has improved in the past 6 years, disclosure of the child's HIV status to anyone in the school might result in possible fear and hysteria and possibly prejudice the child's education. This should therefore be done only with the informed consent of the parents and age-appropriate consent of the child. Should special education services be required, these usually can be done without revealing the diagnosis. A successful AIDS education program should reassure teachers about the nature of the disease and improve the environment so that the school staff can feel comfortable with educating an HIV-positive child should the diagnosis become known.

There are now treatments available for HIV infection, such as orally administered zidovudine (AZT), which may need to be administered during the school day. These treatments should be given in the manner developed for all children who require medication while in school. Since the nature of the medication may identify a child as HIV infected, only those intimately involved with the administration of the medication in school need to be informed. In these cases, this would be only the school medical advisor and the school nurse. The decision for this limited disclosure should be made by the parents and the physician.

Reaction to the disclosure of HIV status may result in discrimination for children with HIV infection in school. Teachers should take the lead in discouraging this by educating students about tolerance of children with chronic illnesses. The pediatrician can play a role in educating parents and the community and discouraging discrimination by utilizing the assistance of public health authorities, American Academy of Pediatrics statements, and the help of religious leaders and others in the community.

Employees

Staff members infected with HIV generally should be allowed to stay at school or on the job as their state of health permits. They should seek the advice of their physicians as to attending work/school. The school policies covering the employment of HIV-infected personnel should prohibit discrimination.

Pupil Needs

A child with HIV symptomatic infection should be regarded as a chronically health-impaired child. School personnel need to be oriented toward the needs of this child. Health services should be available in the school. Special education should be provided as needed under Public Act 94-142 and, for children from birth to age 3, under 99-457. The physician should participate actively as a member of the team. Due to intercurrent illnesses, children with HIV infection may be absent from school frequently and may require occasional home instruction. This should be provided as quickly as possible upon authorization of the team. The child's physician, together with school nurse, should facilitate the transition between school and home instruction.

Health-Related Therapy

Children with symptomatic HIV infection may demonstrate visual, spacial, and perceptual dysfunction. Neurologic findings, including poor fine-motor coordination, clumsy rapid alternating movements, or abnormal gait, have been demonstrated in many such children. These children also may need occupational therapy, physical therapy, and/or speech or language help under appropriate medical supervision.

Behavioral Aspects

Children with HIV infection may present behavioral problems such as anxiety, depression, anger, and withdrawal. These may be due to the neurologic effects of the disease or to the problems associated with family disruption and the resulting parental isolation, guilt, and alienation. Physical changes, such as weight loss and declining cognitive function, may lead to additional emotional problems during the middle school years. The family should be given support by school mental health personnel, and the pediatrician should work with the school and the family in order to provide behavioral counseling and support.

Universal Precautions

Because all infected children will not necessarily be known to the school and officials, policies and procedures should be developed in advance to handle incidences of bleeding because blood is a possible source of contagion. Washing exposed skin with soap and water is the most important preventive measure in this setting. Lacerations and other bleeding lesions in school should be managed in a manner that minimizes direct contact of the caregiver with blood. Under no circumstances should the urgent care of a bleeding child be delayed because gloves are not immediately available. Since many infectious agents may be transmitted by other body fluids such as urine, stools, vomitus, tears, and nasal or oral secretions, hand washing is recommended.

Health Education

The American Academy of Pediatrics believes that AIDS education should be part of a comprehensive school health education program. This should be taught from kindergarten until 12th grade with a planned, sequential health curriculum. During the early elementary grades, a regular, trained teacher is sufficient; however, at the middle and high school level, a qualified health educator should be appointed to supervise AIDS education. Programs might be started during the high school years but then expanded downward to the elementary grades and kindergarten. Finally, parental involvement should be actively encouraged. Parents can obtain AIDS education themselves from schools, community resources, local public health departments, and their own pediatrician.

The Role of the Pediatrician and/or Family Physician

Physicians have an important part to play in AIDS education because of their role as a case manager for children with chronic illnesses, their opportunity to communicate with parents, their knowledge about family structure, and their participation in community affairs. The role of physicians in AIDS education is to begin educating themselves about AIDS. In Connecticut, it was found that the best way of training office physicians in private practice was to train physicians and their office staff together. This was done in six regional areas and took place during a single 3-hour course given in the early evening for physicians, nurses, and all members of their office staffs. Once trained, physicians and their staffs can be effective in promoting school-based AIDS educational programs as well.

The AIDS education programs in schools should be advocated for and supervised by a school health advisory committee or similar school-related organization in each community. This committee may con-

sist of a school medical advisor, community pediatrician and/or public health physician, school nurse, health educator, mental health professional, school administrator, faculty member, parent, and community representatives.

The school medical advisor should be instrumental in educating physicians and nurses in the community. Once trained, they would then: (1) conduct education programs for teachers, parent groups, and other personnel; (2) assist schools and organizations in developing educational programs; (3) review, adapt, and develop education materials; and (4) participate in media events and in discussions between administrators, faculty, and parents.

Physicians can review videocassettes for content and developmentally appropriate levels. They also can participate in review of curriculum materials to make sure they are medically correct and timely. Broadcast media, radio and TV, also are appropriate media for discussing the nature of HIV disease. Physicians may participate in hotlines about the topic or do television interviews. Printed media also may be appropriate vehicles to discuss the subject with parents. Networking is an important aspect of AIDS education. Organizations such as Parents of Children With Chronic Diseases, AIDS support groups, and health education coalitions are appropriate organizations to involve.

Legislation to outlaw discrimination toward HIV patients, both at a local and national level, should be supported. Mandatory testing should be discouraged and voluntary testing supported. Financial support should be provided for the many difficulties faced by parents with HIV infection.

Conclusion

The pediatrician must network effectively with parents and public health authorities in order to ensure the educability of HIV-infected children in school and the education of other children about this disease.

Resources

Pediatricians frequently seek information about AIDS education for use as school medical advisors, for networking purposes, or for their own information and use in their offices. There are now several excellent sources to access. These include the CDC National AIDS Clearinghouse, the CDC National AIDS Information and Education Program (NAIEP), the National Pediatric HIV Resource Center at the Children's Hospital of New Jersey, the National

School Boards Association, the Council of Chief State School Officers Comprehensive Health Education Network (CHEN), and the National Association of State Boards of Education.

The CDC National AIDS Clearinghouse

This clearinghouse is a comprehensive information center for people working in HIV and AIDS, including public health professionals. The center operates information services, distributes materials, facilitates networking, and operates NAC ONLINE. One can call the clearinghouse toll free at 1/800/458-5231. Specialists will answer inquiries and make referrals and help locate publications. They can access the following computer data bases in order to put the caller in touch with organizations providing materials:

The Resource Data Base contains a description of more than 16,000 organizations providing HIV-related services and resources.

The Educational Materials Data Base provides a collection of information on more than 9,000 hard-to-find HIV-related educational materials.

The AIDS School Health Education Data Base is produced by the CDC Center for Chronic Disease Prevention and Health Promotion, Division of Adolescent and School Health. This was developed in 1987 to help organize the various educational resources available to teach children and youth about AIDS and HIV infection. In order to access this combined health information data base, one should call 1/800/289-4277. Use one's own computer terminal and obtain a subscription to BRS, a communications soft package and a modem. (AIDS School Health Information Data Base Maxwell On-line BRS Information Technology Division, 1200 Route 7, Latham, NY 12110.) The data base publishes a manual with a list of references in alphabetical order (audiovisuals, books, brochures, journal articles, etc). The manual also contains a description of the 1989 Cooperative Agreements giving the addresses and phone numbers of national, state, and local programs in AIDS education and national training programs. If you need more information about the School Health Education Data Base or wish to submit materials or information related to AIDS Education, contact the CDC at the Centers for Disease Control and Prevention, Center for Disease Prevention and Health Promotion, Division of Adolescent and School Health, Mail Stop 814, ATTN: AIDS School Health Education Data Base, Atlanta, GA 30333.

The Funding Data Base describes funding activities for community-related HIV and AIDS service organizations. It includes information about application processes, deadlines, and eligibility requirements.

One can obtain materials from the Clearinghouse such as selected reprints from the CDC's *MMWR* and the *HIV/AIDS Surveillance Reports*.

The Clearinghouse also works with national, state, and local organizations and with a number of minority, adolescent, and women's organizations in order to provide exchange about HIV- and AIDS-related services.

Finally, the Clearinghouse operates NAC ONLINE, which is a computerized information network facilitating information exchange among AIDS service providers.

National AIDS Information and Education Program (NAIEP)

This program is responsible for informing the American people about the HIV virus and AIDS. This includes a media communication effort and national information hotline and clearinghouse for the public. The public information aspect creates and promotes "America's response to AIDS" information materials. This is the largest federally sponsored health campaign in history. The CDC National AIDS Hotline operates around the clock, providing anonymous, confidential information in English (1/800/342-AIDS); information also available in Spanish and for the deaf. Trained specialists answer questions about HIV and AIDS. They also work with the National Partnership Development activity that works with private sector organizations to encourage their participation.

National Pediatric HIV Resource Center

This is located in the Children's Hospital of New Jersey, 15 S 9th St, Newark, NJ 07107; telephone number 1/800/362-0071. The center provides consultation and technical assistance to programs serving children with HIV infection, promotes development and distribution of educational materials for patients and family, provides technical assistance on legal issues facing providers, as well as educational opportunities for professionals including an HIV core curriculum. This is an in-depth theory and clinical curriculum for pediatric HIV professionals, including physicians, nurses, and social workers. Mini-fellowships at the Children's Hospital are designed to enhance providers' clinical skills. Workshops are given on ethical and cultural issues as well as "train the trainer" workshops for pediatric professionals to utilize within their own communities.

Interested pediatricians should contact Carolyn Burr, the coordinator, or Dr Samuel Grubman, who is a coordinator of medical education and arranges the clinical training experiences (Telephone: 201/268-8251).

National School Boards Association

This educational organization maintains an HIV and AIDS resource data base that enables policy makers and educators to make informed decisions about HIV and AIDS policy in educational issues. These provide information about AIDS-related issues important to school officials. Pediatricians may want to utilize this source to help discover worthwhile AIDS education curricula to utilize in schools. The data base contains more than 600 entries including resources such as sample policies, curricula, court decisions, books, journals, and videotapes. School officials are encouraged to submit policies and other relevant materials for inclusion and request data base searches to aid in decision making involving HIV and AIDS education policies. The data base may be accessed by calling the National School Board Association, 1680 Duke St, Alexandria, VA 22314 (703/838-6754).

Comprehensive Health Education Network (CHEN)

The Council of Chief State School Officers is funded by the CDC to create a computer network, entitled "The Comprehensive Health Education Network" (CHEN), which enables state education agencies, local education agencies, and national organizations funded by the CDC to share information about HIV/AIDS education and other related issues. Users can also exchange private messages and post information. Users of this data base are able to share and request information about a number of topics, including source materials, curriculum assessment, and policy issues in education. One can also reach select groups of health educators. Those requesting further information may contact Martha Bush, (202/336-7031). Council of Chief State School Health Officers, 1 Massachusetts Ave, NW, Suite 700, Washington, DC 20001-1431.

National Association of State Boards of Education (NASBE)

A useful policymaker's guide to help in planning effective state programs about AIDS education has been published by this association. Entitled *Effective AIDS Education*, the guide can be obtained from the National Association of State Boards of Education, 1012 Cameron St, Alexandria, VA 22314. The National Association of State Boards of Education also has published an *HIV/AIDS Education Survey*, which profiles state actions in each individual state. These publications contain materials, highlights of state policies and programs, and state health education requirements in each of the 50 states.

AAP Provisional Committee on Pediatric AIDS

In 1986, the Academy issued a statement entitled "School Attendance of Children and Adolescents With Human-T Lymphotrophic Virus 3, Lymphadenopathy Associated Virus Infection," which was the first statement on HIV infection in school children and complemented a CDC statement issued earlier. The statement stated that children could attend school on a case-by-case basis and that routine screening for children with HIV infection was not indicated. This paper now is retired and has been replaced by a newer policy statement that includes recommendations listed below. It was of value primarily in that it served to reassure the nation and provide impetus for successful AIDS education programs.

In the course of the need to develop policy and better educate pediatricians about HIV infections, the Academy appointed a Task Force on Pediatric AIDS in the summer of 1987. The Task Force—now a Provisional Committee—meets three times a year and consists of pediatricians with experience in infectious disease, HIV infections, adolescents, perinatal AIDS, foster care, psychosocial issues, disability issues, and school health.

In 1988, the AAP Committee on School Health issued a policy statement entitled, "AIDS Education in Schools," which was reviewed by the Provisional Committee. Recommendations are similar to those described by the CDC and have been described earlier in this chapter. The statement was in agreement with the CDC position that all schools should develop a comprehensive AIDS education program to include children from kindergarten through 12th grade. It recommended that all physicians, especially pediatricians, provide leadership by encouraging development of local AIDS education programs.

In November 1988, the Provisional Committee on Pediatric AIDS published a statement entitled "Pediatric Guidelines for Infection Control of HIV Virus in Hospitals, Medical Offices, Schools, and Other Settings." This report attempted to differentiate high-prevalence areas from low-prevalence areas and provided further reassurance to the public concerning HIV infection control. The paper stated that:

1. Children with HIV who are old enough to attend school could be admitted freely to all activities, to the extent that their health permits.
2. Because all infected children would not necessarily be known to school officials in high-prevalence areas, and because blood was a potential source of contagion, policies and procedures should be developed in advance to handle instances of bleeding. Because of minimal risk, the only mandatory precaution should be washing exposed skin with soap and water. In schools in high-prevalence areas, access to gloves should be provided for those individuals wishing to further reduce the risk; especially if they will be involved in handling of body fluids.
3. Even in high-prevalence areas there is no need for separate examining rooms or visiting rooms for HIV-infected patients, unless the patient is sufficiently immunosuppressed to require reverse isolation.
4. Needles should be placed uncapped in closed puncture-proof containers, which then should be disposed of as infectious waste.
5. All children could be admitted to school and to day care if their health, neurologic development, behavior, and immune status were appropriate.

This paper served as a foundation for subsequent statements on HIV infection and freed physicians from their concern about contagion.

A list of current statements developed by the AAP Provisional Committee on Pediatric AIDS is included below. Also listed are AIDS-related statements developed by other AAP committees. The reader is referred to the Academy for updated information.

AAP Policy Statements

Guidelines for Human Immunodeficiency Virus (HIV)-Infected Children and Their Foster Families
Perinatal Human Immunodeficiency Virus (HIV) Testing
Education of Children With Human Immunodeficiency Virus Infection
Pediatric Guidelines for Infection Control of HIV (AIDS Virus) in Hospitals, Medical Offices, Schools, and Other Settings
Perinatal HIV Infection (AIDS)
Acquired Immunodeficiency Syndrome Education in Schools
Human Immunodeficiency Virus (AIDS Virus) in the Athletic Setting

Suggested Readings

American Academy of Pediatrics, Committee on Children With Disabilities, Committee on School Health. Children with health impairments in schools. *Pediatrics.* 1990;86:636-638

American Academy of Pediatrics, Committee on School Health. Administration of medication in schools. *Pediatrics.* 1984;74:433

American Academy of Pediatrics, Committee on School Health. Concepts of school health programs. *AAP News.* December 1985

American Academy of Pediatrics, Committee on School Health. Guidelines for urgent care in school. *Pediatrics.* 1990;6:999-1000

American Academy of Pediatrics, Committee on School Health. Medically indicated home, hospital, and other non-school based instruction. *AAP News.* February 1992

American Academy of Pediatrics. *Proceedings From a National Conference on Public Law 99-457; Physician Participation in the Implementation of the Law.* Elk Grove Village, IL: American Academy of Pediatrics; 1988

Belman AL, Diamond G, Dickson D, et al. Pediatric AIDS neurologic syndrome. *Am J Dis Child.* 1988;142:29-35

Burger JE, ed. *Responding to HIV and AIDS.* Washington, DC: National Education Association, Health Information Network; 1992

Centers for Disease Control. Education and foster care of children infected with HTLV III/LAV infection. *MMWR.* 1985;34:517-521

Epstein LG, Sharer LR, Oleske JM, et al. Neurologic manifestations of human immunodeficiency virus infection in children. *Pediatrics.* 1986;78:678-687

Majer LS. HIV-infected students in school: who really does "need to know"? *J Sch Health.* 1992;62:243-245

Sklaire MW. Role of the pediatrician in school health. *Pediatr Rev.* 1990;12:69-70. Commentary

Ultmann MH, Belman AL, Ruff HA, et al. Developmental abnormalities in infants and children with acquired immune deficiency syn-drome (AIDS) and AIDS-related complex. *Dev Med Child Neurol.* 1985;27: 563-571

Zlotnik JL. AIDS: helping families cope. Recommendations for meeting the psychosocial needs for persons with AIDS and their families. *Rep Nat Inst Ment Health.* 1987